BASIC HAIRDRESSING

a coursebook for Level 2

SECOND EDITION

Stephanie Henderson
Cert Ed, LCGI

Stanley Thornes (Publishers) Ltd

First published in 1991 by:

Stanley Thornes (Publishers) Ltd
Ellenborough House,
Wellington Street,
CHELTENHAM
GL50 1YW
England

Second edition published in 1995

96 97 98 99 00 / 10 9 8 7 6 5 4 3

British Library Cataloguing in Publication Data

A catalogue record of this book is available from the British Library

ISBN 0–7487–2238–6

Also by Stephanie Henderson:
Hairdressing and Science (Stanley Thornes 1989)

Cover photograph by R. Meredith
Hair by Uxbridge College Artistic Team
Make-up by Jane Kenny

Typeset by Columns Design Ltd, Reading, Berks
Printed and bound in Great Britain at TJ Press Ltd, Padstow, Cornwall.

Contents

Update

This simple practical text book has been completely updated for the revised NVQ/SVQ Level II City and Guilds/Hairdressing Training Board qualifications.

It now also includes these new topics:

- Portfolios.
- Afro hair structure, hair products, hair pressing, curly perms, relaxing.
- Lowlights.
- Colour correction.
- Teamwork.
- Stock control.
- The latest Health and Safety Acts.
- Fashion setting.
- Long hair.
- Barbering techniques (including beards and moustaches).
- Shaving.
- Health matters – fitness for hairdressers.

Introduction

Hairdressing is much more than being able to pick up a pair of scissors. You will need to develop lots of different practical skills such as styling, colouring and perming to produce an individual hairstyle for your client, making them want to return to you again and again. There is always a reason why everything is done a certain way in hairdressing, such as the way the hairdressing scissors are always held with the thumb and third finger so that you can cut the hair at every angle. This basic knowledge is known as the 'theory side' of hairdressing. Once you understand this knowledge you can explain your techniques to other hairdressers and to your clients, should they ask.

This book explains in simple, practical terms what you will need to know to become a good, competent hairdresser. It starts with client care and works through consultation, hair disorders and diseases, selling skills, shampooing and conditioning, blow drying, cutting, perming, relaxing and neutralising, colouring and bleaching, reception, team work, stock control, health and safety, setting short and long hair, and men's barbering and shaving techniques. It is particularly suitable for anyone taking the City and Guilds/Hairdressing Training Board Level II NVQ (National Vocational Qualification) as it covers all the core units, both optional units – setting and barbering – and one additional unit – men's shaving.

Always remember that the most important person is the *client*; salons cannot exist without them! Clients will visit the salon for a variety of reasons:

- They want to *look good* by benefiting from professional hairdressing services, such as
  - cutting, either to create a new style or to reshape the same one
  - perming, to create volume or bounce in the style
  - colouring, to achieve a lighter or brighter colour or blend in a few grey hairs
- They want to *feel good* by relaxing in a pleasant atmosphere, feeling that they are in safe hands because the hairdressers are properly trained.

There are several different types of client – regular, occasional or new – but all of them must be treated with respect, courtesy and pleasantness *every* time they enter the salon. Good communication skills are vital – have you ever been put off from using a certain shop because the staff were miserable and unhelpful? Therefore, you will need to become an expert hairdresser *and* a good communicator to keep your clients.

Clients today are very well informed from the media (television, radio and magazines) and will often ask about the hairdressing products being used on their hair. You will need a thorough knowledge of hairdressing chemicals and equipment and why some are better than others – especially if they are expensive!

People are attracted to hairdressing salons in a variety of ways, sometimes by advertising or press features, sometimes by word of mouth but often by the appearance of the salon. A clean, bright and tidy shop with an attractive reception area and smiling, efficient staff often encourages new customers to enter. Remember, the more clients you have the more successful the salon will be.

Salons can be extremely varied and are not only found in the high street. They can be within:

- large department stores
- cruise liners
- hotels
- health farms
- clinics
- health and fitness clubs
- gymnasiums and leisure centres
- clients' homes (if the hairdresser is mobile)
- hospitals
- residential homes
- holiday camps
- the armed forces.

A career in hairdressing can progress in many different directions – from being a famous hairstylist such as Vidal Sassoon or Trevor Sorbie to owning your own salon or working in the film or television world.

Hairdressing trainees, salon apprentices and full-time college students take the City and Guilds/Hairdressing Training Board Level II NVQ Certificate as their qualification. If you wish to progress from that level you can then train for the City and Guilds/Hairdressing Training Board Level III Certificate, which includes fashion cutting, dressing long hair, specialist colouring and perming, client consultation, demonstrating hairdressing skills and supervising and training staff.

Here are some examples of the many and varied careers available in the hairdressing world.

Film, television and theatrical work

You will need extra qualifications in wig making and make-up, plus some more practical experience with local theatrical companies. There are very few openings: the BBC, for instance, have thousands of applicants for only one or two places. You will also need to be prepared to work all sorts of strange hours when you are needed.

Managerial work

Once you are a qualified stylist you can progress to become a style or artistic director, an educational director, manager or manageress or a salon owner.

Working for a manufacturer
Manufacturers (such as Wella or L'Oreal) employ:

- sales representatives – who sell products to hairdressers
- technical representatives – who give technical advice on products
- demonstrators – who demonstrate hairdressing products in salons, training centres, colleges or within the manufacturers' own schools.

Teaching
Once you are an experienced stylist you can progress to teaching in colleges or training centres, but you will need an advanced qualification such as the City and Guilds/Hairdressing Training Board Level III and a recognised teaching qualification. There are also Skills Assessor and Vocational Assessor awards for those who wish to assess a trainee's practical work.

Trichologist
Hairdressers often refer clients with hair and scalp disorders to a doctor or a trichologist. A trichologist is a hair and scalp specialist who deals with various problems such as hair loss. It takes several years to qualify through the Institute of Trichologists. Once qualified, you can work in either a hair clinic or a hairdressing salon.

It is often said that you never stop learning in hairdressing. You have chosen one of the most interesting, exiting and demanding careers around – enjoy the book and enjoy your hairdressing career!

Acknowledgements

The authors and publishers would like to thank the following for permission to reproduce material:

BLM Health – colour photographs of pediculosis capitis (eggs) between pages 20 and 21

First Direct – 141

Joshua Galvin – 176, 178

Goldwell – colour photographs of smooth cuticles and damaged cuticles between pages 20 and 21, 73

Institute of Trichology and the International Association of Trichologists – photos of psoriasis, alopecia areata, trichorrhexis nodosa, pediculosis capitis (head louse) and folliculitis between pages 20 and 21

Lloyds Bank – 141

L'Oreal – 47, 127

Paul Mitchell – 40

Neville Daniel (hair by Errol Douglas) – 62, 92, 93

Redken Laboratories Ltd – photograph of monilethrix between pages 20 and 21, 104

St. John's Institute of Dermatology, London – colour photographs of tinea capitis (ringworm) and impetigo between pages 20 and 21

Salon Publicity (Giannini Studios) – 183

Simon Spearing Inc – 67 (bottom)

Tondeo – 190

Wella (Great Britain) Ltd – colour photograph of fragilitis crinium between pages 20 and 21, 81, 84, 100, 109, 123, 146, 150, 180, 182, 186, 189, 191, 192, 193, 205, 209

- 81 (left): hair, Keith Harris for Wella; photography, Iain Philpott
- 81 (right): hair, Patricia Dixon of Classics Hair & Beauty of Kenilworth; photography, Alistair Hughes
- 180: hair, Samantha Fox of Martin Gold, Stanmore
- 182: hair, Martyn Maxey at Max & Co; photography, Alistair Hughes
- 186, 191: hair, Kerry Hayden, Wella Studio London Creative Team; photography, Bonieventure
- 189, 192, 205 (top): Wella Studios Manchester – Stuart Kirkham
- 193, 209: Wella Studios
- 205 (bottom): hair, Kerry Hayden, Wella Studio London Creative Team
- colour photographs between pages 196 and 197: Kerry Hayden of Denise McAdam for Wella

Many thanks to hairstylists Gary Lee and Kevin Duigenan of Uxbridge College for cutting and styling photographic work.

Thanks to advisors Brian Smith for Barbering and Shaving; Kirsten de Bouter and Peter Dedes of 'Under Pressure' for Health Matters; and David Brown for technical assistance.

The author and publishers acknowledge the Hairdressing Training Board as originators and copyright owners of the NVQ occupational standards for hairdressing.

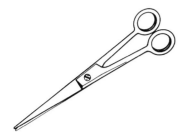

Portfolios

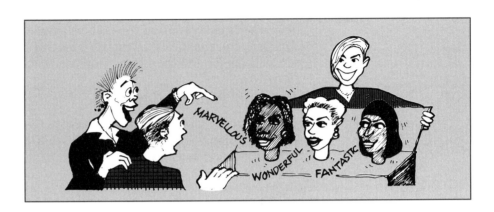

What is a portfolio?

Your portfolio is a collection of both the **work** that you can do **now** (e.g. photographs of the blow-drys you have done) and of **work** that you may have done in the **past** (e.g. a diploma from a manufacturer's hair colouring school). The intention is to show that you can do your job well.

This work that you collect is called **evidence**, and is a necessary part of gaining your **qualification** and **certificates**.

You will normally need a large ring binder file to keep all your (A4) sheets of evidence. Paper sheets are best kept in clear plastic envelopes with small sticky labels (for numbering and indexing later) stuck to the top outside corners.

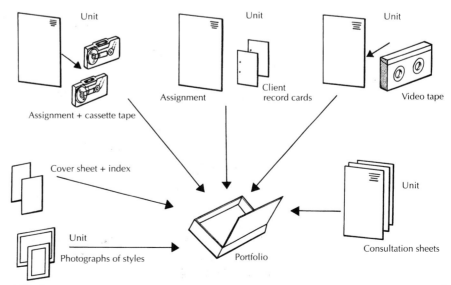

A box file may also be useful for keeping any video or cassette tapes or other pieces of evidence.

Section cards in your file are particularly useful to keep each area, such as your personal information, index system and each unit of work separate.

What should your portfolio contain?

A cover sheet

This should give details of your centre (name, address and telephone number), the qualification (e.g. HTB/C&G NVQ Level II Hairdressing) you are working for and your name (and candidate number, if known).

Personal information

Only include what is relevant to the award (your certificate) – e.g. your job description if you are working in a salon, or a personal account (you may have experienced working with the public within paid or voluntary work).

People involved in the assessment

You should include the names of people who train, assess or verify your work.

A unit checklist

This is often provided by your centre and is completed as soon as you finish each unit, to check your progress.

An individual action plan

This is provided by your centre to help you to know how much and what evidence you will need to provide for each unit and if you will need any further training.

An index

This will be a description of how you have organised your work, for example:

- P1   Cover Sheet
- P2   etc.
- P3   Unit checklist
- P4
   ↓   etc.
- P30   Photo of a bob cut (Ref. A)
   ↓   etc.
- P69   Video of a perm wind (Ref. B)
   ↓   etc.
- P85   Client record card for colouring (Ref. C)

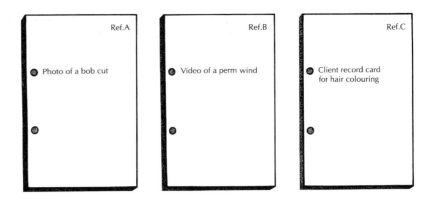

Portfolio index examples

Unit evidence

The unit evidence will contain:

- records of **observation** by your **assessor** (e.g. someone has watched and recorded you shampooing)
- records of any **oral questions** asked by your assessor (these may be recorded on cassette tape)
- products of your **performance**, e.g.
    - **photographs** or **videos** of hairstyles you have produced (try to include yourself in the photo)
    - **client record cards**
    - **consultation sheets** or reports about your work
    - **memos** (recording that you have correctly taken telephone messages)
    - any other **relevant** information such as letters, drawings or computer printouts
- **evidence from other people**, such as letters or reports from managers, other members of staff, clients or other observers (these are called witness testimonies). Alternatively, you could complete your own report or **work log** or **diary** and ask your witnesses to sign it
- **certificates** – e.g. colouring or perming diplomas from manufacturers' schools
- **supplementary evidence** such as projects, assignments, simulations, case studies or records of oral question which cover any gaps in your evidence. This will ensure that you have covered the range (all the work).

All your evidence must be

Valid – it must **relate to the standards** (what is written in your assessment book).
Authentic – it must be what **you**, and **no-one else**, have done.
Current – it must show that you **can currently** do the work.
Sufficient – there must be enough evidence to prove that **you have covered all the work** in your assessment book.

Do's and Don'ts

Do:
- **ask your trainer** or assessor if you need help
- constantly look at your assessment book to **check the requirements**
- **ask others** to help provide **witness testimonies**
- use **illustrations** or **photographs**
- **cross-reference** wherever you can – e.g. use the same set of photographs for cutting, perming and conditioning

- **explain things clearly**, using simple terms and step-by-step techniques
- **present your portfolio in a professional manner** – it must be legible and readers should easily be able find what they are looking for.

Don't:
- make your work any **longer than it needs to be**
- **leave** any areas **uncompleted**
- **lose or mislay any work** – you might have to do it all again!

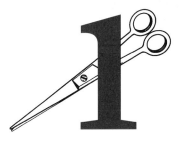

Client care procedures

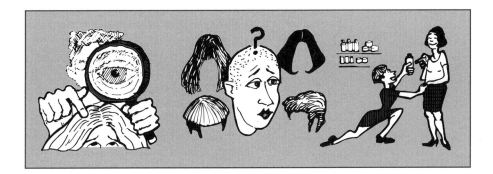

Client consultation means talking to your client and giving advice **before** starting work on their hair.

During this consultation you will also be examining your client's hair by brushing it through. In the same way that doctors diagnose their patients' illnesses, you will be able to diagnose any hair or scalp conditions and take the appropriate action.

You will also be able to assess the client's requirements generally, and make recommendations for a hairstyle to suit their appearance and lifestyle.

Remember

Clients may have no idea of what they want. This is your opportunity to make recommendations and to build up a good relationship, which may lead to a return visit

HEALTH MATTERS

Standing all day long

Shoulders Work with your shoulders relaxed. Exercise helps by contracting and relaxing the muscles. Try raising your shoulders by lifting them up towards your ears and letting them drop. It is possible to do six of these in ten seconds, so try to do it at least twice a day.

Gaining information

Remember

All salon **records are confidential** – those kept on a computer are covered by the **Data Protection Act 1984** – and must not be accessed without your supervisor's permission.

You must find out:

- the client's name
- the service (e.g. cut, perm, colour) required
- the chosen hairstyle (you may need to use a style book).

Record keeping

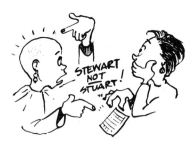

Why bother to keep client records?

- A new stylist will be able to attend to a client **when the normal stylist is away** (off sick or on holiday).
- It is possible to check **when the client last visited** your salon for a colour or a perm (some salons send out reminder cards).
- Clients feel they are being **professionally treated** when they see you are checking their personal records.
- You are able to know exactly what **perm** lotion at which strength and what curler size was used on previous occasions (especially useful if the perm was too tight or too soft).
- You are able to know what make of **colour or bleach** was used on previous occasions, which colour was used, the peroxide strength and the length of time the hair took to process.
- Any **conditioning treatments** recorded will allow you to know how many were needed before the hair returned to good condition.
- You can keep details of any **special conditions**, such as any medication the client has been taking, or details of a resistant section of hair.
- You can deal with any **complaints** more efficiently. For example, if a client complains that a perm has not lasted, but your records show that the perm used was a very soft perm which was only intended to last six to eight weeks, you can remind the client of the details.
- You will have a record of the client's **telephone number and address**, which may be needed if an appointment has to be changed.

Records are generally kept for perming, hair colouring and bleaching, and for conditioning treatments.

Record cards

These are stored either in a filing box or in a filing cabinet, in alphabetical order according to the surnames of the clients.

Cards must be filled in and filed back in alphabetical order after use.

Some salons design their own record cards; others buy or use specially made cards.

Client name						Special notes	
Address							
						Homecare sales	
Daytime telephone no.							
Date	Stylist	Scalp condition	Hair condition	Technique	Products	Develop-ment time	Result

To do

Watch a senior person in the salon:

- finding a client's record card
- completing a record card after a service and returning it to the file.

When the salon is not busy:

- ask about any abbreviations you have not seen before – for example, 30 vol. H_2O_2 means '30 volume strength hydrogen peroxide'
- look through the record cards and make a list of ten clients who have both perms and hair colour.

Computers

Many salons now use computers, not only for recording all the takings but also for keeping client records. You will have to be trained to use it properly. All computers are operated by a program, which is known as the software. Salon computer software will need to classify, store and retrieve information: the type of software used to do this is known as a **database**.

Once all the client records are on the database, then retrieving the information is quick and easy.

Client consultation

Remember

All consultations are done on dry hair before shampooing. You cannot always see the problems (e.g. dry ends) when the hair is wet.

To do

- Watch and note how the stylists in your salon perform a consultation.
- Practise talking politely to clients about their hair.
- Practise making a mental note of the height, size, face shape, age, personality, lifestyle and occupation of your clients.

Experienced hairdressers will be able to produce a perfect hairstyle for each individual client by considering:

- face shape (oval, round, long or square)
- approximate height (tall or short)
- approximate size (thin or overweight)
- approximate age (not everyone can take young styles)
- skin colour
- lifestyle (busy people want a hairstyle that is quick and easy to manage)
- personality (quiet and shy or lively and outgoing)
- occupation (some professions may have strict rules about hair length)
- cost (make sure a price list is accessible)
- medical history (some illnesses affect perming and tinting)
- occasion (dinner dance, wedding)
- time available (can the client spare the time for a long process such as perming?).

NB All this should be done **before** gowning up the client so that you can consider their clothes and lifestyle, and see their height and body shape more clearly.

Talking to clients

Your communication skills are just as important when working with new clients as they are with regular clients. Smiling at others encourages good humour and a pleasant manner. It is very difficult not to smile back at someone who smiles at you.

Look at your client in the mirror or face to face. Eye contact can express friendliness and trust, showing that you are paying attention.

Listen to your client. Many clients never return to a salon because, although they have been given a lovely new hairstyle, it was not the one they asked for!

Speak to your client and explain any reasons for delays straight away, and in a polite manner. Always be **honest** and **factual**. If the client is rushed for time or appears rather cross then ask your supervisor to help.

Remember that a satisfied client is good for business. **A happy client will tell a few people about you, an unhappy client tells everyone.** Clients have every right to expect the service they agreed to have and have paid for.

Test your knowledge

1 Describe why it is important to communicate effectively with your client.
2 All client consultation checklists and record cards are confidential. Why is this important?

Gowning up

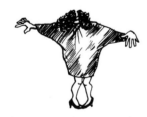

Ideally the stylist will always carry out a consultation with the client before gowning up, so that the client's clothes and lifestyle, height and build can be observed beforehand. Always check with the stylist **when** they would like you to gown up a client.

Gowning up is necessary to protect:

- the client's **clothes** from becoming wet, from falling hair clippings, perm lotion, colours and bleaches
- the client's **eyes and skin** during chemical processes such as perming, neutralising, relaxing, colouring and bleaching.

Gowns

Gowns should always be freshly laundered and tied securely. Some salons use different coloured gowns for different purposes – for example darker gowns (sometimes plastic) for colouring, perming or bleaching.

To do

Watch your supervisor gowning up a client in preparation for:

- shampooing
- cutting
- perming
- hair colouring
- bleaching.

Towels

Clean towels should be used for every client and must be placed securely around the client's neck. They are to be used within the salon for shampooing and chemical processes. Some salons use two towels: one around the front and one around the back, whilst others secure the ends of one towel with a butterfly clamp. Again, check the colour of towel to be used – darker ones are often used for colouring.

Cotton wool strips

Many salons use these to protect the client during perming and neutralising so that the lotion does not run onto the client's skin or into their eyes. The strip is usually dampened with water before being applied so that the perm lotion or neutraliser is not absorbed into the cotton wool strip from the hair.

Neck strips

These are placed between the towel or gown and the client's neck to prevent any hair clippings or chemicals falling on the client's clothes.

Remember

Always check that the client has removed large earrings, other jewellery (e.g. necklaces) or glasses if necessary before gowning up. Ask the client to keep them in a safe place (in a bag for instance).

Make sure you tuck the client's clothing inside the gown, especially high-necked jumpers.

Barrier cream

This is carefully placed around the client's hairline (*not* on the hair) to prevent skin being stained by colours or to protect sensitive skin during bleaching or relaxing. Sometimes barrier cream is placed on the scalp as an extra protection during chemical relaxing.

Cutting capes

These are usually plastic and are placed around the shoulders during cutting so that the hair falls easily from the cape.

Examining the hair and scalp

Finding out what the client wants to have done to their hair and choosing a style is very important, but sometimes the hairdressing service possible depends entirely on what the client's hair and scalp condition will allow.

For instance, if the hair is untreated it means that no chemicals have been used on it, but if it has been chemically treated it will react differently to blow-drying and setting, perming, colouring and bleaching.

HEALTH MATTERS

Standing all day long

Legs   Many hairdressers suffer from varicose veins, especially if they have had children. This is because you are not moving your legs when you are standing still and the blood does not circulate properly back to the heart. The result can be both swollen ankles and varicose veins (because the veins have become full of blue, deoxygenated blood).

If it is impossible to take a rest at work with your feet up, make sure that you do it at home by raising your feet on a stool or another chair.

Exercise is the best way to prevent varicose veins. If you cannot walk or cycle to work, then try doing it in the evenings or on your days off. Walking is an excellent form of exercise.

A temporary colour (a coloured mousse or setting lotion) affects different parts of the hair than does a permanent colour (a tint). You will need to recognise the different parts of the hair and learn how they are affected by various chemicals, and whether coloured hair can be permed, coloured or bleached in future.

Hair can be damaged by chemical treatments. It can also be damaged by handling – bad brushing, excessive blow-drying or tonging. Again, you will need to know what part of the hair is damaged and whether further services can be carried out.

As you are carrying out your consultation you can start to diagnose your client's hair condition. In order to understand why some people have shiny, manageable hair in good condition but others have very difficult hair you need to know more about hair structure.

Hair structure

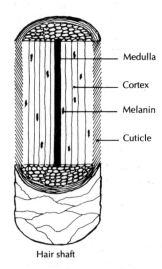

Medulla

Cortex

Melanin

Cuticle

Hair shaft

Longitudinal section of a hair

Each hair is made up from three layers – in a similar way to a pencil.

- The outside layer, the **cuticle**, is thin and flat (like the paint on a pencil).
- The middle layer, the **cortex**, is the strong, main part of the hair (like the wood of the pencil).
- The central layer, the **medulla**, runs finely through the middle (like the lead in a pencil).

The cuticle

If you look carefully at the diagrams you will see that the cuticle is actually made up of **overlapping scales** (7–10 layers). These scales look like the tiles on a roof, with the edges of the scales all lying away from the scalp. They are translucent, like frosted glass, so that the hair colour (in the cortex) can be seen through them.

This outside layer of the hair shaft is very tough and holds the whole hair together, but it may be damaged by strong chemicals (such as perms or bleaches) or harsh treatments (such as over back-brushing).

Once the cuticle scales have been damaged or broken and have opened up, and chemicals have been absorbed into the cortex, the hair surface will look and feel rough and dull (like sandpaper). If the scales are undamaged and closed tight and flat then the hair will appear beautifully shiny (like glass).

The cortex

The cortex is the main part of the hair, lying underneath the cuticle. Hairdressers need to understand the cortex because this is where all the changes take place when the hair is blow-dried, set, permed, tinted and bleached.

It is made from many strands or fibres, which are twisted together like knitting wool. These can stretch, then return to their original length.

Hair is made of a protein called **keratin**, itself made up from amino acid units, which are found in long coiled chains called **polypeptide chains**. All the coils of polypeptide chains are held together by various links and bonds.

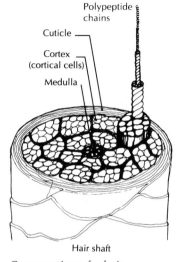

Cross-section of a hair

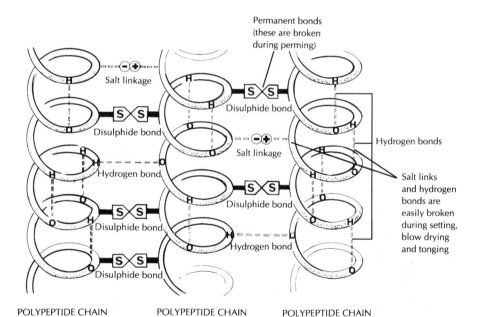

The structure of keratin

Look at the diagram above and find the **temporary bonds**. These are the **hydrogen bonds** and **salt links**. They break and rejoin wherever hair is blow-dried, set, tonged or hot brushed into a different style. They are called temporary bonds because all of these processes are easily reversed by dampening the hair and starting again.

There are also **permanent bonds** in the diagram: these are called **disulphide bonds**. Disulphide bonds are very strong and can be broken only by using a strong chemical such as permanent wave lotion on the hair.

The cortex also contains all the **colour pigments** in the hair. These pigments are called **melanin** (brown/black) and **pheomelanin** (yellow/red).

The medulla

The medulla does not really have any real function. It is not always present in scalp hairs, particularly if the hair is fine.

To do

- Sketch the diagram of the hair structure and label it (without looking at your book).
- Make a list of all the technical words related to hair structure that you have just learned and explain them in your own way.
- Copy the diagram of the structure of keratin, then try to draw in and name the links and bonds (without looking at your book).

Scalp (or skin) structure

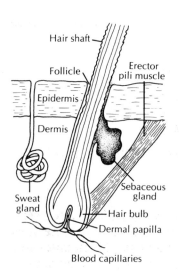

Structure of the skin

There are two main types of hair on the human body. Fine **vellus hair** grows on the body and stronger **terminal hair** grows on the scalp (and makes up eyebrows, eyelashes, beards and moustaches). A third type of hair, **lanugo hair**, is only found on human foetuses and is even finer than vellus hair. The scalp is stronger than the rest of the body skin (which is why we can put chemicals on scalp hair without causing too much damage) but its structure is otherwise similar to body skin.

Hair is made of the protein keratin, which is dead. There are no nerve endings inside hair and so it does not hurt when we cut through it, or when chemicals such as perm lotions or bleaches are put onto it.

However, we can feel someone pulling our hair because it is attached to the scalp by its root, sitting in a tiny pocket called the **hair follicle**. Nerve endings attached to the hair root tell us when our hair is being pulled and when a hair should stand on end. We all have occasional 'goose pimples', the hair standing on end if we are very cold or frightened. The **arrector pili** muscle is attached to the hair root and contracts (or squeezes together) to pull the hair upright, creating the goose pimples.

The **sebaceous gland** is also attached to the hair follicle and produces **sebum**, the hair's natural oil or lubricant. The sebum flows around the hair root and outwards onto the scalp surface. If too much sebum is produced the scalp and hair are too greasy, but if too little sebum is produced the hair and scalp are too dry.

The scalp (and skin) is divided into two layers:

- the outer layer – the **epidermis** – is the outer protective layer of skin. It is constantly shedding itself, losing dead skin cells. When this happens excessively on the scalp it is known as dandruff
- the inner layer – the **dermis** – is the thickest and most important part of the skin. It is where the hair follicles, nerve endings, sebaceous glands, blood supply and sweat glands are found.

Hair could not grow without its own blood supply. Our hearts pump blood containing food and oxygen (needed to make new keratin) through our arteries towards the skin surface. The arteries become **small blood capillaries** in the dermis, where they feed blood into the bottom of the hair root or follicle to feed the dermal papilla. The more blood there is flowing towards the hair papilla the more the hair will grow. Therefore, when our skins are red and warm in the summer our hair (and nails) grow quicker.

We can also regulate our body temperature through our skin because we have **sweat glands**. These produce sweat which flows on to our skin through our pores, cooling us down when it evaporates.

To do

■ Copy the diagram of the scalp and skin structure and then try to label it up on your own.
■ Describe the structure of the scalp or skin in your own words.

Ethnic structural hair types

There are three main racial differences in hair types:

● European hair – **Caucasian** – is generally wavy
● Asian Hair – **Mongoloid** – is usually straight
● Negroid Hair – **Afro-Caribbean** – is usually curly

Each type of hair will react differently to different hairdressing processes.

Afro hair structure

Afro hair is naturally dark because it contains **more melanin**. It also needs **more care and conditioning** than Caucasian (European) hair because of its curly and crinkly shape. It tends to tangle easily, and may be damaged and break at the ends simply by being disentangled with combs and brushes.

Its curl is formed because of **uneven keratinisation**. This means that the keratin in the hair is **more dense** on the inside of the curl or wave – the **'para'** cortex – and **less dense** on the outside of the curl or wave – the **'ortho'** cortex.

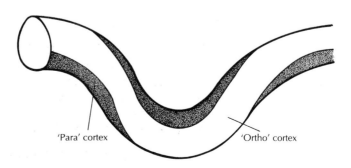

'Para' cortex   'Ortho' cortex

Afro hair structure

Afro hair has slightly **more cuticle** layers than Caucasian hair and is therefore **initially more resistant to chemical processes** such as tinting, bleaching, perming and relaxing. Because it has more cuticle it has **less volume of cortex**, and once chemicals have entered through the cuticle and into the cortex they will **process afro hair more quickly** than Caucasian hair.

Hair thickness

This is known as **hair texture**, and is determined by the thickness of each individual hair – whether it is coarse, medium or fine.

 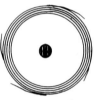

Very fine hair   Average hair   Very coarse hair

> **Remember**
>
> Some people have very fine hair, but lots and lots of it, while some people have very coarse hair but not very much of it.

> **To do**
>
> - Pull out three hairs from your head: one from the front, the middle and the back.
> - Ask several friends to do the same.
> - Compare the thickness of each individual hair against a sheet of paper.

Hair growth and life cycle

Hair grows from the bottom of its root at the dermal papilla, where new cells are constantly being produced. These soft cells become hardened to form strong hair above the skin surface. The average rate of hair growth is 1.25 cm ($\frac{1}{2}$ inch) per month. This amount of hair growth keeps hairdressers in business!

> **To do**
>
> Look again at the typical growth rate of hair. Work out how often you should recommend your client to return for:
>
> - cutting
> - perming
> - highlights
> - permanent hair colouring.

There are approximately 100,000 hairs growing on the average scalp, and there is a constant daily loss of 50–100 scalp hairs. We lose these hairs because every so often the hair follicle has a period of rest, and so the hair falls out.

The growing stage of the hair is called the **anagen** stage. When the hair starts to go into its resting state, it is said to be in the **catagen** stage. The resting stage is called the **telogen** stage.

Obviously not all hairs rest at the same time – or else we would go bald!

> **Remember**
>
> The word ACT:
> A = Anagen
> C = Catagen
> T = Telogen.

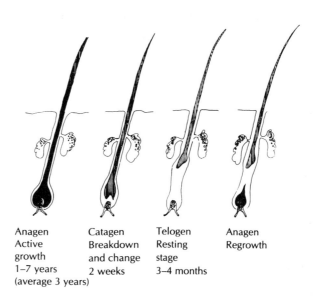

Anagen	Catagen	Telogen	Anagen
Active	Breakdown	Resting	Regrowth
growth	and change	stage	
1–7 years	2 weeks	3–4 months	
(average 3 years)			

Hair growth life cycle

This diagram shows how the hair gradually stops growing and starts again.

Each hair grows for between $1\frac{1}{4}$ and 7 years before reaching a resting stage. This means that some clients' hair will grow to shoulder length:

$1\frac{1}{4}$ years $\times$ 1.25 cm ($\frac{1}{2}$ inch) per month = 18.75 cm ($7\frac{1}{2}$ inches)

but other clients' hair will grow down to their waist or longer:

7 years $\times$ 1.25 cm ($\frac{1}{2}$ inch) per month = 105 cm (42 inches).

So when a client complains that they cannot grow long hair you can explain to them that it is because their hair has a short life cycle.

> **Test your knowledge**
>
> 1 State a typical growth speed for hair.
> 2 Copy the hair growth life cycle diagram and try to label it without your book.
> 3 Explain in your own words why hairdressers need to know about hair growth life cycles.

Abnormal hair and scalp conditions

These may be

- **non-infectious** – they cannot be spread from one client to another, for example **alopecia** (baldness).
- **infectious** – they can be spread from one client to another, for example **head lice**.

Non-infectious hair and scalp conditions

Although a non-infectious or non-contagious disorder may appear unsightly, it **cannot be spread** from one person to another and **can be treated in the salon**.

For illustrations of non-infectious diseases, see the colour photographs between pages 20 and 21.

Non-infectious diseases and conditions of the hair and scalp

Name	Description	Cause	Treatment
Pityriasis capitis (dandruff)	Small, itchy, dry scales, white or grey coloured	Overactive production and shedding of epidermal cells Stress related	Anti-dandruff shampoos Oil conditioners or conditioning creams applied to the scalp
Seborrhoea (greasiness)	Excessive oil on the scalp or skin	Overactive sebaceous gland	Shampoos for greasy hair Spirit lotions
Fragilitis crinium (split ends)	Split, dry roughened hair ends	Harsh physical or chemical damage	Cutting and reconditioning treatments
Damaged cuticle (tangled hair)	Cuticle scales roughened and damaged, hair dull	Harsh physical or chemical damage	Reconditioning treatments Restructurants
Trichorrhexis nodosa (swollen, broken hair shaft)	Hair roughened and swollen along the hair shaft, sometimes broken off	Harsh use of chemicals (e.g. perm rubbers fastened too tightly during perming) Physical damage (e.g. from elastic bands)	Restructurants Recondition and cut hair where possible
Monilethrix (beaded hair shaft)	Beaded hair (a very rare condition)	Uneven production of keratin in the follicle	Treat this hair very gently within the salon
Psoriasis (silver scaling patches)	Thick, raised, dry, silvery scales often found behind the ears	Overactive production and shedding of the epidermal cells. Possibly passed on in families, recurring in times of stress	Medical treatment Coal tar shampoo
Alopecia areata (round bald patches)	Bald patches	Shock or stress. Hereditary	Medical treatment High-frequency treatment
Male-pattern baldness (baldness, thinning hair)	Receding hairline, thinning hair	Genetic or hereditary baldness	Medical treatment is being developed
Cicatrical (scarring) alopecia	A permanent bald patch where the hair follicles have been destroyed	A scar from skin damage caused by chemicals, heat or a cut	None
Sebaceous cyst (lump on scalp)	A lump either on top of or just underneath the scalp	Blockage of the sebaceous gland	Medical treatment

Infectious hair and scalp conditions

Infectious or contagious disorders **must not be treated in the salon.**

Deal with the client sympathetically and tactfully. Explain that you have found a certain hair or scalp condition, which means that you cannot continue with their hair service. You must then recommend that the client **seeks medical advice** from either a doctor or a trichologist (a specialist in hair and scalp disorders)

All **equipment** must be **cleaned and sterilised** after contact with such a condition (see Chapter 10).

For illustrations of infectious diseases, see the colour photographs between pages 20 and 21.

Infectious diseases and conditions of the hair and scalp

Disease	Description	Cause
Pediculosis capitis (head lice)	Highly infectious Small, grey **parasites** with six legs, 2 mm ($\frac{1}{12}$ inch) long, which bite the scalp and suck blood. The female insects lay eggs called 'nits' which are cemented to the hair Very common in children	Infestation of head lice which lay eggs producing more lice living off human blood Treatment is by using special shampoos or lotions containing either Malathion or Carboryl
Tinea capitis (ringworm)	Highly infectious Pink patches on the scalp develop into round, grey scaly areas with broken hairs It is most common in children	**Fungus** Spread by direct contact (touching) or indirectly through brushes, combs or towels
Impetigo (oozing pustules)	Highly infectious Blisters on the skin which 'weep' then dry to form a yellow crust	**Bacteria** entering through broken or cut skin
Folliculitis (small yellow pustules with hair in centre)	Small yellow pustules with hair in centre	**Bacteria** from scratching or contact with an infected person
Warts (small raised lumps)	Small flesh-coloured raised lumps of skin	**Virus** Spread by direct contact: touching. These are infectious only when damaged

Test your knowledge

1 Describe each infectious and non-infectious condition and its cause, without looking at your book.
2 List which hair and scalp conditions can be treated in the salon.
3 Describe the treatments that are available for the conditions that can be treated in the salon.
4 List the conditions that must be treated by a doctor.

Establishing hair condition

Hair in good condition will shine and look great. Clients with a new haircut and hair in good condition will also find that perms, colours and highlights take equally well.

However, hair that is damaged and dry may need special perm lotions or different types of colorants to improve the condition.

Internal and external hair condition

Location	Good condition	Poor condition
Surface condition	Cuticle scales lie flat and close together Surface is smooth and shiny	Cuticle scales are raised and open, sometimes damaged Surface is rough and dull, e.g. fragilitas crinium (split ends) Damaged cuticle This is known as **porous hair**
Internal condition	The chemical links and bonds in keratin within the cortex are strong and elastic and contain natural moisture	The chemical links and bonds in keratin within the cortex have been broken by strong chemicals, e.g. perm lotion, hydrogen peroxide. This hair has lost strength, elasticity and moisture (through the open cuticle scales). It is known as **over-elastic hair** (stretchy hair)

Test your knowledge

1 List the indicators of hair in good condition.
2 List the indicators of hair in bad condition.

Physical and handling damage

Here are some causes of physical and handling damage:

- **bad brushing** – disentangling from the roots instead of starting at the ends
- **bad combing** – over back-combing.
- **over-drying** – the hairdryer too hot and held too close to the hair
- excessive use of **electrical appliances** – tongs and hot brushes
- **excessive tension** – especially from rubber bands
- **strong sunlight**, **sea** and **chlorinated water** – hair lightens and dries out
- very **windy conditions** – cause hair to tangle.

Chemical damage

You already know what chemically damaged hair looks like but you need to know some of the reasons why the damage may have happened. For instance, a perm could look straight either because it was over-processed (a straight frizz) or because it was under-processed. The under-processed perm could possibly be repermed but the hair of an over-processed perm would be sure to disintegrate and break off if further perming was attempted.

The general reasons why hair may be chemically damaged are:

- clients have used products from the chemist **without any professional skill** or knowledge
- the hairdresser has not carried out a **proper consultation** or analysed the hair thoroughly
- the hairdresser has **misinterpreted** the client's requirements
- the hairdresser did not have enough **practical skill, product or technical knowledge**
- the product was **applied badly**, left on too long (over-processed), or not long enough (under-processed).

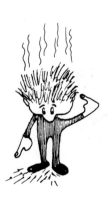

Remember

Physical or handling damage is caused by bad brushing and combing (over back-combing) or excessive drying (hairdryer too hot, excessive tonging or hot brushing).
   Weather damage is caused by excessive exposure to the sun, sea and wind.
   Chemical damage is caused by excessive perming, bleaching (highlighting) and tinting.

Some specific reasons for chemical damage are:

- **perming** – hair looks frizzy and may break off (the scalp may be sore or burned)
- **relaxing** – curly hair has been permanently straightened and is starting to break off
- **bleaching and highlighting** – hair looks and feels 'straw like' and the colour may be patchy
- **tinting** (tint applied on top of tint) – the hair feels very dry and the colour is patchy and uneven
- **colour strippers** – hair may be patchy in colour if strippers are not applied quickly and evenly.

Test your knowledge

State the effects of incorrect application of:

1 bleaches
2 tints
3 perm lotion
4 neutralisers
5 colour strippers.

To do

- Collect as many cuttings of hair in good and poor condition as you can find in your salon.
- Stick them down on paper and caption each with possible reasons for the condition.

Designing a hairstyle to suit your client

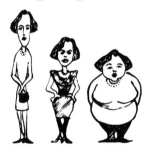

Have you ever wondered why two clients with exactly the same colour, texture and length of hair and the same hairstyle look quite different? It is not only because of their height and build but also because of their head, face or neck shape. Clients must be advised according to these limitations.

Head shape

The shape of a person's head can be clearly seen when the hair is wet and combed flat against the scalp. If the head is flat on the crown for instance, you can compensate for this by leaving the hair longer in that area during cutting.

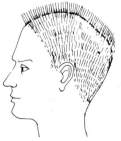 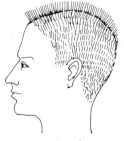

Head shapes for 'flat top' hairstyle

Bad   Good

Head shapes can also look quite different from the front just by altering the parting from side to centre. A side parting will make the head appear broader and wider; a centre parting will make the head appear narrower and thinner.

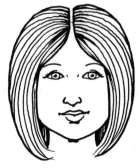 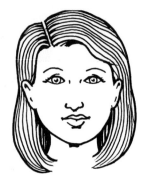

Face shapes

There are four main face shapes: oval, round, square and oblong (long).

Oval

An oval face shape is ideal and suits any hairstyle.

Round

Round faces need **height** to reduce the width of the face. A straight centre parting will also help to reduce the width.

Square

Square-shaped faces need round shapes with wisps of hair on the face to soften them and give the illusion of being oval.

Oblong

Long faces suit short, wider hairstyles dressed around the sides of the face. A low side parting will also make the face look wider.

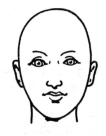

Oval

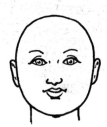

Round

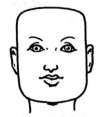

Square

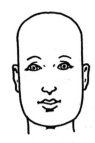

Oblong

To do
■ Comb all your hair away from your face when it is wet and try to decide on your own face shape.
■ Make notes on your consultation sheets of different clients' face shapes.
■ Check with your supervisor to see if these are correct.

Neck shapes

Long and thin necks are more apparent with short hairstyles, and so need longer hair around them. Short necks can be made to look longer by an unswept or flicked style.

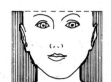 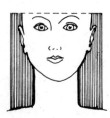 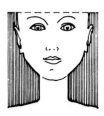

Ear shapes and levels

Generally, large ears, or even large lobes, are highlighted by hair cut short or dressed away from the face. It is better to leave the hair longer over the ears.

Some clients have ears that are uneven, so *never* balance a haircut by the level of the ears.

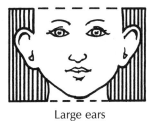
Large ears

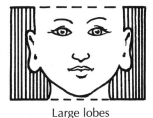
Large lobes

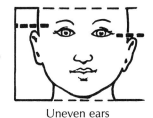
Uneven ears

Nose shapes

A large nose will be more obvious from the side view when hair is drawn back from the face, whereas dressing the hair forward helps to minimise it.

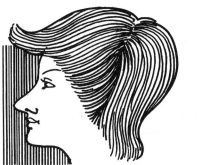
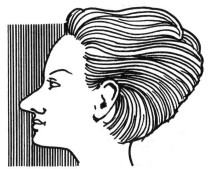

Body build and height

One of the main reasons for consultation with the client **before gowning up** is so that you can briefly judge their body build and height.

Smaller clients can look overwhelmed by too much hair, or made to appear shorter from the back by wearing their hair too long.

On the other hand, large or overweight clients need a style with some volume and length to create a balance between their heads and their bodies. Short, flat hairstyles can highlight large bodies.

Age

A client's age is always an important consideration. Sometimes it is difficult to judge how old a person is, but generally softer styles with more movement are flattering on older people. Avoid straight angular shapes.

Older clients also lose colour tone from their skin, so very few have naturally rosy cheeks; any redness is often caused by broken veins or cosmetic make-up. Dark or ashen colours can therefore be very ageing on older clients who, wishing to look younger, may want to return to the natural hair colour of their youth. Unfortunately this does not always suit them as they get older.

Client lifestyles

The client's lifestyle, occupation and personality is very important

Lifestyle
The client could be a young working mother, who will not have much time to spend on her hair.

Occupation
For example the armed forces and catering professions, which have strict rules about the length of hair.

Personality
A quiet, shy person might not be as daring with new styles as an outgoing extrovert. Clients are often worried about other people's reactions to a new hairstyle, and may say 'I'm not sure if my husband/wife will like it.'

Style books
Style books are very useful. They can be bought from hairdressing suppliers, or you can make your own. You can then adapt any of the ideas you have from the pictures to suit your **individual** clients.

To do

Make your own style book:

- buy a plastic folder with clear plastic inserts to hold cut-out pictures of different styles
- illustrate the front cover with your salon's name and logo and **your name**
- organise the style book in sections – e.g. short styles, long styles, styles to show hair colours, styles to show different types of perms, styles for special occasions (parties or weddings), styles to suit different face shapes.

Hair growth patterns

Hair movement means the **amount of curl or wave** already in the hair, but **hair growth patterns** means the **direction** in which the hair falls.

This natural fall can best be seen on wet hair. If you comb your client's hair back from their face and gently push the head with the palm of the hand you can see the natural parting falling between the front hairline and the crown.

If you are cutting an all-one-length hairstyle such as a classic 'bob' then you must cut it to the natural parting. Otherwise, when the client tries to do their hair at home, the style could hang unevenly with long ends straying down.

There are several unusual hair growth patterns.

Double crown

If the hair is cut too short on the crown it is impossible for it to lie flat - the hair must be left longer.

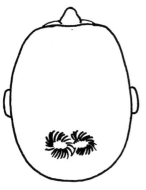

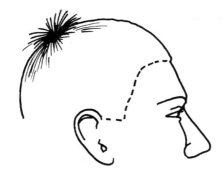

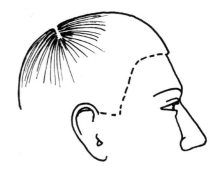

| Double crown | Unsuitable – crown cut too short | Suitable – longer crown hair |

Cowlick

This is found at the front hairline and makes straight fringes on fine hair difficult to cut. It is better to sweep the hair to one side.

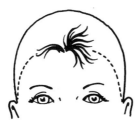

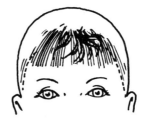

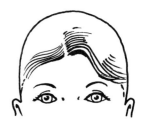

| Cowlick | Unsuitable for full fringe | Suitable for uplift fringe |

Nape whorl

This type of hair growth pattern makes straight hairlines difficult to achieve. It is better to cut the hair short into a 'V' shape or grow it longer so that the weight of the hair holds it down.

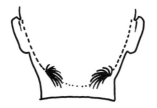

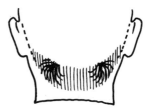

| Nape whorl | Unsuitable for short straight nape | Suitable for 'V' shape nape |

Widow's peak

This is where the hairline grows forward at the front to form a strong centre peak. It is difficult to create a full fringe because the hair tends to separate and lift.

It is better to style the hair back off the face or create a very heavy fringe so that the weight of the hair helps the fringe to lie flat.

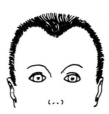

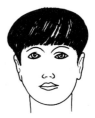

Explaining hair treatments to clients

Once you have decided on the type of hairstyle to suggest to your client you should **explain it in simple terms**. If you went into hospital to have an operation, the doctor would explain what was going to happen to you in clear non-technical language to make you feel much more confident about what is going to happen to you.

Some clients also feel quite anxious about certain hair treatments such as perming or colouring and need reassurance.

If you explained a conditioning treatment as a 'cationic, deep-acting chemical which is substansive to the hair, penetrating deep into the cuticle layers and helping to reduce the hair's ability to absorb atmospheric moisture', the client may become somewhat confused!

However, if you said 'I'd like to apply some of our own deep-acting conditioner to your hair to help the dry, flyaway ends to become shinier and more manageable', the client will understand more about the product and why you are using it.

Hair and skin tests

Whenever you are unsure about how a treatment will turn out you should test the hair first. Hairdressers always use a professional colour chart when selecting a colour so that they do not make mistakes. Testing helps to make both you and the client more confident.

Porosity test

Porous hair can absorb liquids (water or chemicals) through the cuticle and into the cortex.

If the cuticle is closed, flat and undamaged then the hair feels smooth. However, once the hair has been physically or chemically damaged then it becomes generally more porous or unevenly porous. This is why special perm lotions are used for tinted and highlighted hair, as normal-strength lotions could quickly over-process or hair colour could become patchy.

Non-infectious diseases

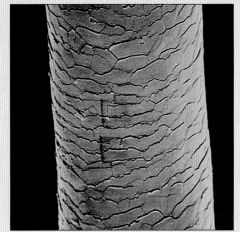

Smooth cuticles

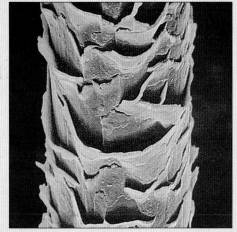

Damaged cuticles

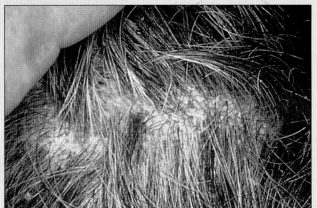

Psoriasis

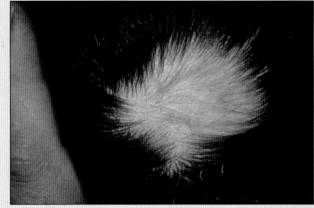

Alopecia areata

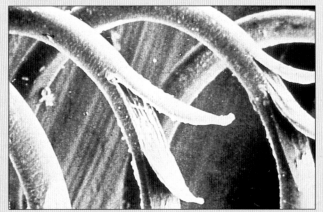

Fragilitis crinium

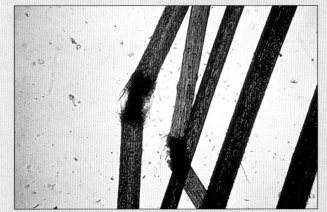

Trichorrhexis nodosa

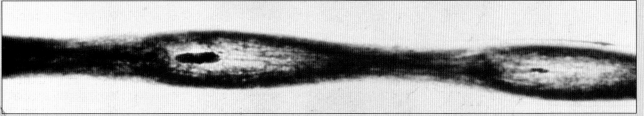

Monilethrix

Infectious diseases

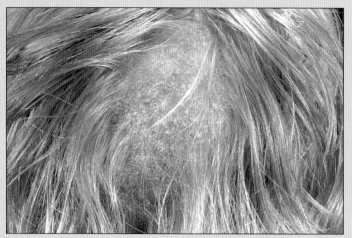

Tinea capitis (ringworm)

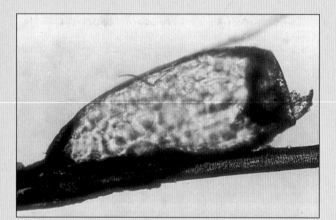

Pediculosis capitis (eggs or "nits")

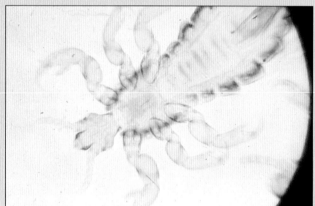

Pediculosis capitis (head louse)

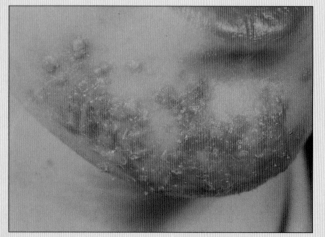

Impetigo

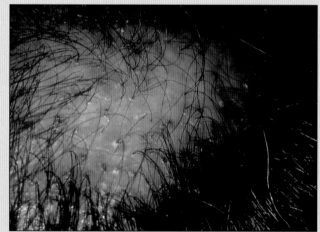

Folliculitis

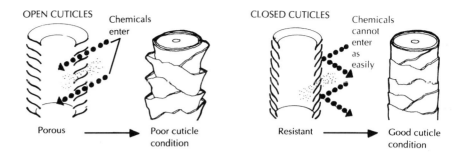

OPEN CUTICLES Chemicals enter

CLOSED CUTICLES Chemicals cannot enter as easily

Porous ⟶ Poor cuticle condition

Resistant ⟶ Good cuticle condition

Porous and resistant hair

Method

To carry out a porosity test, take a few strands of hair and hold them firmly in one hand near the points or ends and slide your fingers along the hair towards the roots. The rougher the hair feels the more porous it is and the more damaged the cuticle scales are.

To do

■ Practise the porosity test on different types of hair.

Elasticity test

Well-conditioned hair is springy and bouncy; this means it has good elasticity. It can stretch up to one-third of its length when dry, half of its length when wet and then returns to its original length.

However, hair that has lost its elasticity because the internal chemical links and bonds in the cortex have been damaged may stretch up to two-thirds of its length or even break off.

Method

To test hair for elasticity, take some dampened hair between your thumb and forefinger and gently pull. If it stretches more than half its length then it is over-elastic and may break off.

To do

■ Watch your stylists testing for elasticity when processing highlights.
■ Ask your supervisor if you may be allowed to test for elasticity under supervision.

Incompatibility test

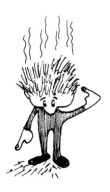

Some products that **clients may have used** on their hair may react badly with some of the chemicals that you intend to use – the hair may go green, steam or break off.

The most common products are **hair colour restorers**, such as Grecian 2000. They contain metallic salts such as lead acetate and the colour develops over a period of time. The hair often looks slightly greenish and feels harsh to the touch. The problem is that most clients do not admit using them because **they do not consider they are colouring** their hair (they think they are **restoring** their natural hair colour).

In the salon a client with hair colour restorer on their hair **must not have**:

- a tint
- a bleach or highlights
- a perm (it is the perm neutraliser that reacts)

because all of these products contain hydrogen peroxide.

If you suspect a client has hair restorer on their hair, carry out an incompatibility test. Some temporary hair colours (colours that wash out of the hair), e.g. glitter sprays, also contain metallic salts and need to be removed.

Method

Mix 40 ml of 20 vol. (6%) hydrogen peroxide with 2 ml of ammonia (perm lotion will do) in a glass measuring container. Cut a few hair samples (use hair affected by metallic salts) from an unnoticeable area of the client's head and secure them with either cotton or sticky tape. Place the hair samples in the solution and keep them under observation. Results could take anything from one to thirty minutes to show.

If the hair has **changed colour**, if **bubbles have formed** in the solution or if the solution has **become warm** then there are definitely metallic salts on the hair.

Do not proceed with any hairdressing process that involves using hydrogen peroxide.

To do

- Visit several chemist's shops and make your own list of all the products available that are similar to Grecian 2000 so that you can remember their names.
- Practise an incompatibility test when the opportunity arises.

Colour test: taking a test cutting

In the same way that you would take a hair cutting for an incompatibility test (from an unnoticeable part of the hair), you can easily test hair to see how it will take a hair colour.

Once the hair cutting is secured by cotton or sticky tape at the ends it can be tested with any of the following:

- **temporary colours** – coloured setting lotions or coloured mousses
- **semi-permanent colours** – colour which last four to twelve washes
- **permanent colours** – tints that are mixed with hydrogen peroxide
- **bleaches** – used for highlights or general lightening.

Method

Mix a small amount of your intended product in a tint bowl and make sure that the test cutting is completely covered with product. Read the manufacturer's instructions to check the development time, but remember that the tints and bleaches will need longer than this to develop, because there is no warmth from the head to make them work.

After the development time, rinse off the semi-permanent, tint or bleach products (temporary colours are left on) and dry the test cutting. With the client, examine it under natural light (near a window) and decide whether both of you are happy with the result.

Test cuttings are also useful to show whether the hair will take the colour evenly, especially if it is unevenly porous.

To do

■ Take test cuttings from white, blonde, medium-brown and dark hair and try them out with samples of your salon products.
■ Attach them to cards and record all the details.

Strand test

A strand test is taken while the following products are on the hair to check when the product has developed thoroughly:

- semi-permanent colours
- permanent colours (tints)
- bleaches
- colour strippers (colour reducers)
- relaxers.

Method
Remove some of the product from a strand of hair with a piece of cotton wool or the back of a comb so that you can see whether it has developed properly, leaving the hair either the correct colour or the correct degree of straightness.

To do

■ Watch your stylist taking strand tests.
■ Ask your supervisor if you may be allowed to take a strand test under supervision.

Pre-perm test curl

This test is taken if the hairdresser is in any doubt about the likelihood of a perm being successful. If the hair is in poor condition (over-porous or over-elastic) it is better to try out a few curlers first, rather than ruining the client's hair.

Method
Either cut a small piece of hair and tie it with cotton or proceed with a small section of hair on the head. Check with your supervisor when choosing the strength of perm lotion and the appropriate size of rollers to use. Wind the hair around the roller, apply the lotion, develop it for the recommended time, then rinse and neutralise.

If the test is carried out on a hair cutting, once the curl is dry it can either be stored away or shown to the client immediately.

Pre-perm test curls are used to:

- decide the **correct strength of perm lotion** to use
- decide the **correct size of perm curler** to use

- determine the **amount of time** the perm lotion should stay on the hair (development time)
- decide whether the hair is in **good enough condition** to take a perm – if in doubt, take an elasticity test.

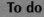

To do

- ■ Read Chapter 5 on perming and neutralising.
- ■ Watch your stylists perming and make a note of the different steps in the procedure.

Development test curl

This test is taken when the perm lotion is on the hair during the development process. Once the curl is fully developed the hair is neutralised.

To do

- ■ A development test curl takes a lot of practice and experience, so watch closely when your stylists are carrying them out.
- ■ Ask your supervisor if you may be allowed to take a development test curl under supervision.

Method

Undo the rubber fastener from one end of the curler. Unwind the curler $1\frac{1}{2}$ turns, without letting the hair unravel completely. Hold the hair firmly, with both thumbs touching the curler.

Push the hair towards the scalp allowing it to relax into an 'S' shape. Do not pull the hair – remember it is in a very fragile state.

When the size of the 'S' shape corresponds to the size of the curler, the processing can be stopped.

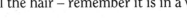

Unwind 1½ turns

'S' shape to size of curler

Taking a development test curl

Test your knowledge

State the purpose of each of the following tests:

1 pre-perm test curl
2 development test curl
3 test cutting
4 porosity test
5 elasticity test
6 incompatibility test
7 strand test.

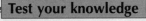

Skin tests

Many people suffer from allergic reactions to food or products (e.g. make-up). Hairdressing is no exception, and clients can become allergic to some hair colours. Permanent colours (which are tints mixed with hydrogen peroxide) and any semi-permanent colours containing para dyes always need a skin test.

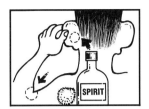

Skin tests must be carried out before each application of the hair colour (usually between 24 and 48 hours before). If the client has a positive reaction (redness, blistering, itching, etc.) para dyes must not, under any circumstances, be used.

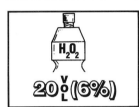

Method
Clean a small, sensitive area of the skin (either behind the ear or in the crook of the elbow) with cotton wool and surgical spirit.

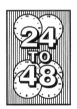

Mix a small amount of the colour to be used with equal parts of hydrogen peroxide, either 20 vol. (6%) or 30 vol. (9%).

Apply a small smear of the colour (about the size of a 20 pence piece) to the cleansed area. Allow to dry naturally.

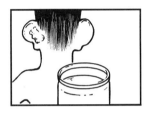

Cover with collodian (New-Skin) and allow to dry.

Ask the client to leave the skin test for 24–48 hours, unless there is any irritation, in which case it should be washed off and calamine lotion applied to soothe the skin.

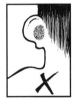

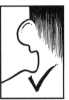

Record which colour and which strength of peroxide you used on a record card, together with the client's name, address and the date.

Check the skin test when your client returns to the salon. A **positive reaction** (redness, soreness, itching or swelling) means that your client is **allergic** to the colour. A **negative reaction** (the skin appears quite normal when the colour is washed off) means that **you can proceed** with the colour.

Remember

Other names for a skin test include patch test, predisposition test, allergy test, Sabouraud Rousseau test, hypersensitivity test.

Test your knowledge

1 State the functions of skin tests in predicting reactions.
2 Describe the visible signs of a positive reaction to a skin test.
3 State the significance of a positive reaction.
4 State the significance of a negative reaction.

Consultation checklists

Once you have read this chapter and understand the variations in client's appearances and hair and scalp conditions you may find the checklist on the following pages helpful for choosing the most suitable products, techniques and equipment to achieve the required look.

General consultation checklist

Consultation and diagnosis for all salon services

To be used for Unit/Element No _____ Formative/Summative

Date_____ Student's name _____ Client's name_____

☐   ☐   ☐   ☐

tick appropriate box

Client requirements

When was the client's hair last shampooed? _____

Scalp condition   Possible disorder/disease _____ Dry/flaky/normal/oily

Hair   **Texture** Coarse/medium/fine   **Volume** Thick/medium/thin

       Type Afro/Caucasian/Asian   **Movement** Straight/wavy/tight curly

       Condition   Normal/naturally dry/resistant

       Previous chemical treatments   P/W/relaxed/tint/highlights/lowlights

       Hair growth patterns   Nape whorl/widow's peak/cowlick/double crown

Testing procedures Elasticity/porosity/incompatibility/strand test/pre-perm test/skin test

Present style   Very long/long/medium/short/very short

               Layered/graduated/one length/club cut/
               razored/clippered/other _____

Client limitations _____

Any additional medical notes _____

Client lifestyle _____

Suggested style _____

Shampoo/surface conditioner recommended_____

Conditioning

Time taken

Name of disorder_____   Product recommended _____

Massage movements _____   Equipment used _____

Cutting

Time taken

With/without fringe   With/without parting   Layered/graduated/one length

Club cut/thinned/razored/clippered/other _____

Time taken [____]	**Styling** Blow-dry description _____ Tools used _____ Finger dry/natural dry Set description _____ Roller sizes _____ Pin curls _____ Styling products _____ Finishing products _____
Time taken [____]	**Chemical treatments** **Perming** Virgin hair/tinted/bleached Pre-condition? _____ If yes, which product? _____ Rod size _____ How many? _____ Winding method _____ Lotion type & strength _____ Processing time _____ With/without heat
Time taken [____]	**Neutraliser** Type _____ Method _____ Conditioning products _____
Time taken [____]	**Relaxing** Product _____ Method _____ Processing time _____
Time taken [____]	**Colouring** Natural hair colour depth _____ % of white _____ Temporary/semi-permanent/quasi-permanent/permanent tint bleaching/lightening Full head/regrowth/partial head Product name and shade no _____ Peroxide strength _____ Method of application _____ Development time _____ Conditioning products _____
Time taken [____]	**Barbering** Beard shape _____ With/without moustache With/without sideburns Presence of male pattern baldness _____
	Additional services recommended to client _____ **Additional products recommended to client** _____
	Client statement Did the stylist discuss with you your requirements before any services began? _____ Was advice given for your hair and scalp care? _____ Did the stylist recommend products? _____ Will you consider following the recommendations? _____ Stylist signature _____ Client signature _____ Assessor signature _____

Sample questions for clients

Here are some examples of questions to ask your clients:

- 'How often do you shampoo your hair?' If the answer is 'every day' then the client probably has greasy hair and scalp.
- 'How have you been lately?' This gives the client a chance to tell you if they are taking any medication that may affect their hair condition.
- 'Do you have your hair permed or coloured?' The client can then tell you about any chemicals they may have used on their hair.

To do

- Make your own list of **tactful** questions to ask the client relating to the consultation checklist.
- Check them with your supervisor.

Ensuring a successful consultation

Remember

Practise communicating – you can only get better!

You will need to win over your client so that:

- he or she comes out with a style which is flattering and their hair in first-class condition
- you do not lose them to the salon down the road!

Here are some helpful guidelines:

- use **colour charts and style books** to explain your points
- **listen** to the client, nodding now and again
- **reassure** the client and be understanding
- offer alternative, **positive suggestions** such as, 'Your hair cannot be permed at the moment but after a series of conditioning treatments, I can perm it in six weeks time'
- **do not use technical language**
- use **eye contact** and **smile** occasionally at the client
- use the **client's ideas** to your advantage, e.g. 'I like your idea of a short haircut, but with your natural hair growth pattern at the front [the client has a cowlick], I could create a great flicked fringe if it was left a little longer there'.

Test your knowledge

1 Describe what could happen if you carried out a consultation incorrectly.

Selling skills

Communicating with people

You can be an excellent stylist but you will never be a successful hairdresser without good communication skills. Clients will return to you again and again if you always do their hair well *and* make them feel special.

Good communication skills when hairdressing include always being polite, cheerful and **listening to the client**. Many clients never return to salons because they have been given a lovely new hairstyle, but not the one they asked for!

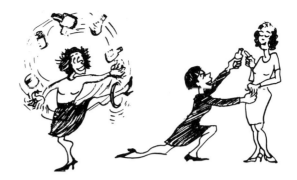

To do

- Read the section on 'Problems can happen' on page 145. Describe to your supervisor how you would cope with a client who had to be kept waiting for an appointment.

If you are worried about chatting to your clients, try to ask questions that are open-ended, such as 'How long have you been coming to this salon?' or 'How do you manage your hair when you go on holiday?' These questions cannot be answered simply by 'yes' or 'no', and so you can start a conversation.

Remember

Never discuss religion, politics, sex or race with clients, as you can easily cause offence and find yourself in an argument.

Try to develop a **sense of tact.** Bad atmospheres can often be created by a slip of the tongue, e.g. 'My goodness, you *do* have bad dandruff'. **Confidentiality** is also important. If one of your clients suffered from head lice, for instance, the worst thing you could do would be to tell any other clients. Not only would these other clients worry that they might catch head lice, but gossip soon spreads and people might become wary of coming to your salon.

Try to increase your general knowledge by reading newspapers or by listening to news programmes on the radio.

Once your confidence is established when dealing with clients, you can start to develop your selling skills.

Explaining various salon services

All the services that are available in your salon will be displayed on the price list. Clients will often ask about the benefits of different services, and by reading this book you will have already increased your knowledge.

Here are some explanations you might give:

- 'Our reconditioning treatments work particularly well because we give a special massage to help them to penetrate into the hair.'
- 'We give two types of permanent waves. One is for a firm curl which lasts well, the other is an acid perm which is gentler on the hair and will not dry it out.'

Here is a fuller description of a client discussion:

Discover client needs

Stylist: 'Your hair has some pretty lightness at the very ends. Is that from your holiday last summer?'

Client: 'Yes, the sun lightened it, but it has nearly grown out now.'

Stylist: 'We could always place some natural-looking highlights through your hair to keep it going until next summer.'

Describe features of service

Client: 'Oh yes, how is that done?'

Stylist: 'By using either cap highlights or foil. The cap method is quicker and less expensive, but the foil gives more highlights exactly where you want them, and you can vary the colour.'

Client: 'What sort of colour would you suggest?'

Look for buying signals

Stylist: (Uses shade cards) 'These light beige blonde tones exactly match the ends of your hair and would look very natural.'

Client: 'How long do they last?'

Describe benefit to client

Stylist: 'They will grow out gradually, and they give your hair a lot more body, which would help your fine hair to keep its style longer.'

Client: 'How much would they cost?'

Close sale

Stylist: 'They are normally £40.00 but we have a special offer for £30.00 if you can make a Monday or Tuesday appointment.'

Client: 'Yes, thank you, I'll make an appointment for next week.'

You can also use style books and product leaflets, rather than just words, to show the client what you mean.

Clients will naturally want to know the cost of the service so make sure you work it out correctly.

It is also important to explain to the client the **length of time involved** for different services. For instance, a short cut and blow-dry with little hair removed may only take 30–45 minutes whereas a restyle, cut and blow-dry for a client with long hair needing to be cut short may take well over an hour.

Remember

Some salon services include the cut and blow-dry (e.g. cut, blow-dry and perm for £45.00), while other services (e.g. conditioning treatments) may not. These will also vary from salon to salon. Check with your supervisor to make sure what is included in each of your advertised prices.

To do

Read the section in Chapter 7 on appointments and make a short list of the benefits, availability, cost and time of the following services:

- cutting
- perming
- colouring
- bleaching
- conditioning
- styling
- consultations.

Retailing in the salon

All hairdressers have an excellent opportunity for selling products in the salon in that they know **what to use** and **how to use** it. Once you have tried your particular salon mousse, for instance, you will understand its benefits (firm hold, non-sticky, gives lift, etc.) and find it easy to explain these benefits to your clients.

To do
Make a short list of each of the products sold in your salon and make a note of: ■ the benefits of each (e.g. normal hold, conditions dry hair) ■ how to use it (e.g. apply to towel-dried hair, apply with your fingertips) ■ the difference between similar products (e.g. conditioners for permed, coloured or naturally dry hair).

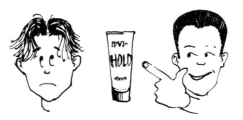

You can show the products to clients by the display at the reception area, but allowing clients to handle products also helps to sell them. If the client can touch, feel or smell the product – especially when you are using it on their hair – you will always gain their interest.

Understanding your market

You will be selling hairdressing services and hairdressing products to lots of different **types of clients**, each having various characteristics – long faces, round faces, high hairlines etc. – which make it important for you to recommend the **correct product**, service and hairstyle for each client.

Here is an example of how to sell a product.

Describe client needs

Stylist: 'Your hair is still a little dry at the ends; would you like me to use our new conditioner today, at no extra charge?'

Client: 'Yes please. What is this one?'

Describe product

Stylist: 'Well, it's one that you actually leave in the hair and don't rinse out. So it does save time.'

Client: 'Won't it leave my hair feeling sticky?'

Stylist: 'Not at all. Try a little on your hands. You can rub it into your skin and see it disappear. It works like that on your hair.'

Client: (Tries the product on her hands) 'Yes, my hands do feel soft and smooth.'

Describe features

Stylist: 'You can use it every time you shampoo your hair and also use it as a hand cream!'

Client: 'How much do I need to use?'

Describe how to use it

Stylist: 'Just squeeze out the size of a small coin, rub the palms of your hands together and smooth the conditioner into the ends of your hair.'

Client: 'Can I buy it at reception?'

Close sale

Stylist: 'Yes, the prices of all the sizes are clearly marked. Remember you get a hair conditioner and a hand cream for the same price!'

Once you have gained some product knowledge, you will find the best way to talk about it is to do it in this order:

1. Describe the product – what it is (e.g. shampoo, hairspray).
2. Describe how it works – what it does (e.g. especially benefits permed hair or hair that is washed frequently, or prevents salon colours from fading).
3. Describe how to use it (e.g. hold the hairspray 30 cm away from your hair, or shake the can immediately before use).

Here are some examples of client types:

- young and fashionable
- professional business people
- students
- young mothers
- senior citizens
- children
- uniformed professionals (e.g. nurses and police officers)
- European
- Afro-Caribbean
- Asian
- Oriental.

To do

- Make a short list of the products and the services that your salon has to offer to suit some of the above client types.
  e.g. young and fashionable – firm-hold mousse, short clippered styles
  senior citizens – regular use of hair spray, firm, curly perms.
- Read the sections on 'Tools and equipment' and 'Electrical appliances' on pages 55–9. Make a list of the best types of tools and equipment your clients should buy to use at home and the correct methods of using them, e.g. brushes, combs, hairdryers and other electrical equipment.
- Re-read the section on designing a hairstyle to suit your client and make notes on which styles suit different client characteristics, e.g. round face, long neck, etc.

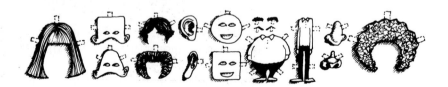

Developing and responding to non-verbal clues

There are other ways of responding to your client as well as talking to them. People communicate **non-verbally** all the time, using both appearances and gestures.

Appearances

Hairdressing is all about creating images. Remember, not everyone wants a new hairstyle whenever they visit the salon. Many clients are quite happy for you to maintain the style they have, with a few possible variations.

Use your common sense when selling services and products. For example, a young working mother with little time to spare would be more willing to buy a combined shampoo and conditioner or a 'wash 'n' wear' perm than would a senior citizen with more time on their hands.

Gestures

The obvious gestures that you should look for when selling products and services are:

Head nodding

This means that a client is listening to what you are saying with agreement. A slow single nod means you should continue what you are saying, and several quick nods mean that the client wants to interrupt and speak themselves.

Eye contact

By looking into someone's eyes you can soon see if they are being friendly or hostile towards you. When you are selling to clients, do look them in the eye while speaking to them to gain their confidence.

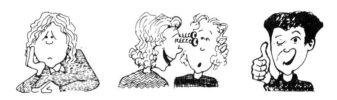

Smiling

Simply occasionally smiling at clients will automatically create good humour in the salon. It is very difficult not to smile back at someone who smiles at you!

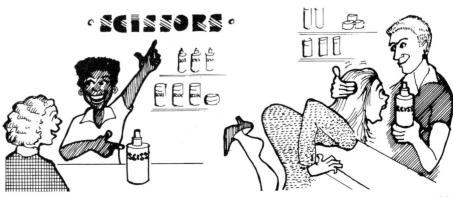

Selling: the three stages

Remember, there are three stages to selling:

1. **Finding out the client's needs** means identifying any previous treatments or problems. You will have learned to do this tactfully during the consultation process. Examples might include fine lank hair, itchy scaly scalp, dry, split ends.

2. **Giving the client advice** means asking any relevant questions that will lead you to suggest a particular service or product. Here are some examples:

   - fine, lank hair – 'Have you ever thought about having a soft body perm which just gives volume and bounce?'
   - itchy, dry scalp – 'Do you find your itchy scalp becomes worse with certain shampoos?' ('We have one which is especially soothing', etc.)
   - dry, split ends – 'How often do you have your hair trimmed? We recommend cutting every six weeks to reduce split ends'.

3. **Gaining agreement with the client** is achieved by either receiving an immediate response or giving them time to think about it. For example, 'Would you like a perm on your hair now?' or 'My hair has been easy to manage with this perm. I'm sure that yours would be too'.

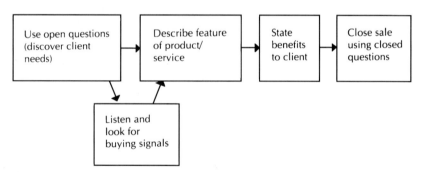

Finally, do not forget to record any sales or client services on your record card for next time.

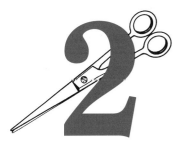

2 Shampooing and conditioning

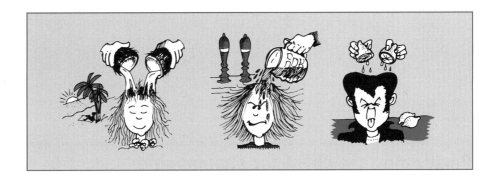

One of the first procedures learned in the salon is shampooing a client's hair. The client is paying for this service so it must be done properly and better than they could do it themselves.

Reasons for shampooing hair

Clean hair makes you feel great, and a thorough shampoo will remove not only dirt and grease but also hairspray, mousse, gel, setting lotion, flakes of dead skin on the scalp and temporary colours (coloured mousse or colour setting lotions). Tints, bleaches and highlights are also removed from the hair by shampooing.

In the salon, hair is shampooed **before** styling – and particularly before perming. This is because hairspray, mousse or conditioner on the hair would form a barrier and prevent the perm from taking.

Gowning up

Remember

You may need to notice what the client is wearing when choosing a hairstyle.

Clean gowns and towels are placed around the client after consultation. Disentangle the hair with a brush or comb at this point. Normally a gown, towel and plastic shampoo cape is placed around the client to protect them from any water seeping down on to their clothes.

HEALTH MATTERS

Many salons now have free-standing shampoo basins where the shampooist can stand upright rather than leaning across to shampoo the client from one side. The free-standing basins are better because your weight is evenly balanced. If you have to stand on one side, then try to work on one side with one client and from the other side with the next client.

During shampooing try to relax your shoulders and keep your elbows down and in towards your body. Keeping your wrists straight during massage will prevent as much strain as possible.

Most salon shampoos are dispensed from large bottles and the shampoo is forced through a small hole. If this hole becomes encrusted with dried shampoo it becomes even smaller and it is difficult for the shampoo to come out. You may have to strain your wrist and forearm by squeezing hard, so clean the nozzle frequently and keep the container full.

Positioning the client for shampooing

Remember

The client should be comfortable, dry and relaxed after shampooing: check to make sure.

Various types of wash-basins are used in salons: back wash, side wash and front wash.

Back wash and side wash basins

The client must be seated comfortably when reclined, with their neck placed centrally in the neck rest of the basin. Most back wash chairs are specially sprung, so when the client leans backwards the back of the chair reclines allowing them to remain comfortable. Do adjust the chair for the client if necessary.

Front wash basins

Tall or short clients, children or people with back problems often require a front wash. Front wash basins are more difficult to use and you must protect the client's face – particularly from any dangerous chemicals you are using near their eyes (e.g. when neutralising perms or removing bleaches). A small hand towel should be offered to the client as a face protection.

Testing the water temperature

Remember

If you accidentally scald yourself with hot water, run **cold** water over the area for 5–10 minutes.

Using the water spray during shampooing takes practice, so test the controls first. Turn on the cold tap first at a moderate rate of flow, then mix in water from the hot tap until the correct temperature is reached. Test the temperature of the water by spraying it either on your wrist or the back of your hand and adjust it as necessary.

Remember

The sensitivity of the scalp to temperature varies from person to person, and what is comfortably warm to one person may be too hot for another, so check that your client is comfortable with the water temperature.

To do

■ Practise turning on the water spray to the correct temperature and testing it on your wrist a few times **before** shampooing your first client

The hardness of the water

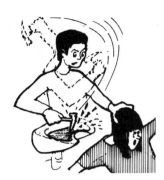

Both water sprays and mixing valves need regular maintenance because **limescale deposits** ('furring up') develop if the water is hard. This can cause blockages and low water pressure, causing hair rinsing to take a long time. Look at the shower spray heads regularly to see if they need cleaning. The head can be cleaned either in place, using a fine pin, or by unscrewing it and using a liquid descaler.

Soft water

If the salon is in a **soft water area**, or uses a water softener, then you will **not** find limescale deposits in water spray heads or 'furring up' in your kettle. Soft water will also lather up easily when you wash your hands with a bar of soap and no scum will be left in the basin.

Hard water

You will know if the water is **hard** in your area because limescale deposits will be formed around your salon spray heads, in the kettle, and in your steamer (if you have one).

Hard water contains dissolved **calcium and magnesium salts** – it is these that produce scum when you wash your hands with soap.

If you have a steamer in your salon it must be filled with distilled water (softened water) so that limescale cannot build up.

To do

■ Wash your hands with a bar of soap in your salon and decide if the water is hard or soft.

General types of shampoo

Remember

Hairdressers do not wash hair with soap; shampoos are **soapless detergents**.

Soap

A bar of soap or a container of liquid soap is used for washing your hands, not your client's hair. This is because scum is formed from hard water salts – imagine the scum that is left in the basin after washing your hands being left in your client's hair!

Shampoo (for use on wet hair)

Shampoos are made from soapless detergents with various additives –

Remember

To avoid shampoo dermatitis:

■ do not wear rings while shampooing
■ rinse and dry your hands
■ use a good hand cream regularly

lemon, coconut, almond, etc. The shampoo combines with any greasy dirt on the hair during lathering. Hair is then effectively cleaned when the shampoo is rinsed from the hair. Soapless detergents are very strong and when you are shampooing regularly in the salon you may suffer from **dermatitis** on your hands.

Dry shampoos

Sometimes it is impossible to wash a client's hair, for instance if there is no hot water (during a power cut) or if the client has a tender scalp after illness. The hair of such clients can be dry-cleaned (like clothes) by using:

- **Spirits** (alcohol) such as white spirit. Pour the spirit on to cotton wool, rub it on to the hair, then rub clean cotton wool (or a clean towel) over the hair to remove the grease and dirt.
- **Dry powders**, which are like fine talcum powder. Sprinkle them on to the hair then brush through, allowing them to absorb grease. Dry powders often leave the hair looking dull, so are rarely used in the salon.

The pH Scale (acidity and alkalinity)

Hairdressing products, especially perm lotions, relaxers, shampoos and conditioners, often have labels relating to pH. Clients often ask 'why is an acid perm better than an alkaline perm?' or 'why do some shampoos leave my hair so dry?' The answers can sound very technical, but it really is quite simple.

The degree of acidity or alkalinity of a hairdressing product can be measured on the pH scale, which runs from pH1 to pH14, where pH7 is neutral, (neither acid nor alkaline). pH values greater than 7 indicate alkaline substances: **the higher the number the more alkaline (and harmful) the product**. A pH value less than 7 indicates acid; **the lower the number the greater the acidity**.

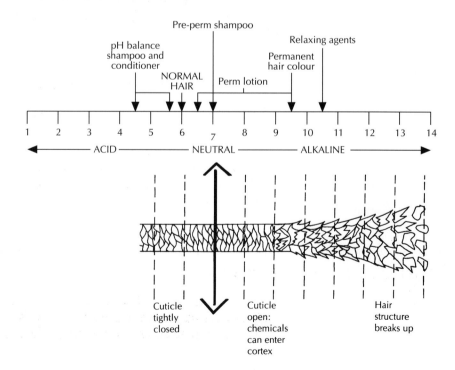

Hair and skin pH scale

The chart opposite shows that the pH of the hair and scalp is 4.5–5.5, which means they are naturally slightly acid. This is why acid-balanced products are better for the hair and scalp.

To do

■ Research as many hairdressing products as you can find in your salon and local chemist shops to find out which products state the pH and what these pH are.

The diagram of the effect of pH on the hair cuticle shows that **acids keep the cuticle scales closed**, so the hair looks smooth and shiny. However, **alkalis open the cuticle scale**s, making the hair look rough and dull. Hairdressing processes such as perming, bleaching, tinting and relaxing are all alkaline because they have to lift the cuticle scale in order to penetrate the cortex and perform their chemical action.

Therefore any conditioning product which has an acid pH (4–6) will leave the hair in a shiny, smooth condition.

The pH of shampoo

Remember that **pure water is neutral** and will not open or close the cuticle scales. Hair is slightly acid (pH 4.5–5.5), so that the cuticle scales are naturally closed.

When you use an **alkaline** shampoo (pH above 7) the cuticle scales will **open**, which is helpful before perming as it allows the perm lotion to enter the hair easily.

When you use an **acid-balanced** shampoo (pH below 7) the cuticle scales will close, which is helpful after bleaching and colouring as it will make the hair shiny again.

To do

Take a piece of litmus paper (which indicates pH acidity and alkalinity) and test:

■ all the shampoos in your salon
■ either a bar of soap or some liquid soap
■ the water you use to shampoo your clients' hair

Choosing the right shampoo

It will be up to you to choose the correct shampoo for the client's hair and scalp type. Always check the manufacturer's instructions – some shampoos have to be diluted and some are left on the hair for a few minutes.

| **To do** |

■ Re-read the sections in Chapter 1 regarding hair and scalp conditions.

Never ask the client which shampoo they want – **you** must explain which shampoo (and conditioner) would be most suitable for them.

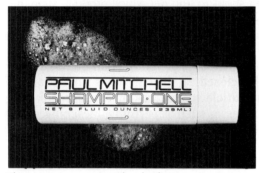

This contains coconut for dry hair

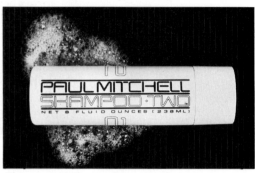

This contains lemon for greasy hair

Hair conditions and shampoo types

Hair condition	Shampoo type
Greasy scalp and hair	Lemon, plain soapless shampoo
Dry scalp with dandruff	Anti-dandruff or medicated shampoo
Naturally dry hair	Coconut, almond or lanolin shampoo
Chemically dry hair (permed, tinted or bleached)	Protein-conditioning shampoo
Fine, flyaway hair	Volumising shampoo
Hair with excessive hairspray	Shampoo with lacquer-removing solvent
Hair about to be permed in the salon	Plain, soapless shampoo with **no additives** (these could form a barrier to the perm)
Hair that has just been tinted or bleached in the salon	Acid-balanced shampoo, pH 4.5– 5.5

Method for shampooing

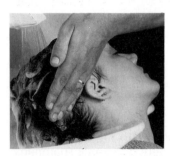

Once you have completed your client consultation, positioned your client at the basin, chosen a suitable shampoo (and conditioner if needed) and tested the water temperature you are ready to start.

Wetting the hair

The hair must always be **wetted thoroughly** by holding the water spray close to the head and directed away from the face following the different angles of the head.

Start at the centre of the forehead, making a barrier with your free hand to protect the client's face from water. Sweep the water over the hair using

Remember

Always turn off the water while you are lathering the shampoo and massaging the scalp. **Save hot water – it is expensive.**

Remember

If you spill any water or shampoo on the floor, wipe it up immediately to prevent anyone from slipping or falling.

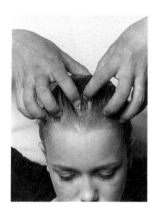

Remember

Only use effleurage on the ends of long, dense hair to prevent tangling.

the spray and hand together. Cup your hand when above and around the ears, patting the water up into the nape hair. Remember to hold the spray until you have turned the water off.

To do

■ Find where the stop-cock is in the salon; you never know when you might have a burst water pipe and need to shut the water off.

Applying the shampoo

Never waste shampoo. Look at the amount of hair the client has. A short head of fine hair needs less shampoo than a thick head of long greasy hair. Use a little shampoo at a time – if you use too much you will have to rinse out a large amount of lather.

Shampoo needs to be applied in several places over the hair, but always pour the shampoo into the palm of your hand first, as this will prevent the shock of cold shampoo on to the client's head.

Massage

Starting at the centre of the forehead by the hairline, push your fingers through the hair to the scalp and begin to massage with the pads of your fingers (not your fingernails).

Do not keep your palms flat, but arch your palms and fingers as though you were grasping a large ball. Open and close the whole hand, keeping your fingers well spread and allow the fingers of one hand to pass between those of the other.

When shampoo is spread on to the hair it is called an **effleurage** massage movement. Once the shampoo is evenly applied to the hair and you are giving a deeper massage – this is known as a **rotary** movement, and helps to thoroughly cleanse the hair. All scalp massage has a beneficial effect in that the blood flow to the skin surface is stimulated, helping to encourage hair growth.

Rinsing

Once you have achieved a good lather, rinse the hair thoroughly until the water runs clear. Check around the front and back hairlines to ensure that no shampoo is left in the hair. Gently squeeze out any surplus water from the ends of the hair.

Applying a surface conditioner

If a surface conditioner is being applied at the basin, place the required amount (the **thicker** and **more concentrated** the product, the less you need) into the palms of your hands and spread evenly through the lengths of the **hair**, **not** onto the **scalp**. Always check the manufacturer's instructions when using any shampoo or surface conditioner as many have to be left on for 3–5 minutes to be effective.

Disentangling

Use a wide-toothed (rake) comb to disentangle the hair, starting at the ends and working towards the roots so that you do not tear the hair. This may be done either at the wash-basin or at the dressing position.

Bringing the client to an upright position

There are many variants in the method of using shampoo towels, but what is really important is that the client should remain dry and comfortable.

Bring the client to an upright position when you are ready by asking them to sit up.

Towel drying the hair

Towel-dried hair is hair that is still wet but does not have water actually dripping from it. Hold the towel in both hands, pressing the hair between the two sides of the towel in a smoothing action. The hair is then ready for further processes.

Variations when shampooing

Before perming
Always use a plain soapless shampoo and do not apply a conditioner before perming as there must be **no barriers** on the hair.

Two-in-one shampoos, which cleanse and condition the hair at the same time, can cause product build-up on the hair and create a **hidden barrier**. If the client has been using this product then you must remove it by using a deep-cleansing **clarifying** shampoo.

After tinting and bleaching
Remember, the scalp will be more sensitive after chemical processing, so **do not massage too harshly** and **do not have the water too hot**.

Tints and bleaches have to be rinsed thoroughly from the hair before it is shampooed, **twice**, to remove all the chemicals. Some tints have a shampoo base in them and will lather up when water is applied.

Shampoos for Afro-Caribbean tight curly hair

Afro hair is much drier than Caucasian (European) hair and shampoo for afro hair contains both mild detergents and higher concentrations of **moisturising** and **detangling** agents, creams or oils. A separate **oil-based conditioner** must always be applied to the **hair and scalp** after shampooing and left on for three minutes before rinsing. Afro hair that has been **chemically treated** and is **badly damaged** needs products containing more conditioning agents that add both **moisture** (i.e. oils such as coconut, which help to retain moisture) and **protein** (such as hydrolysed protein or keratin).

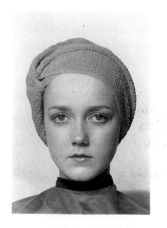

Remember

Semi-permanent colours are always lathered then rinsed out of the hair, **never shampooed** out.

Test your knowledge

1 What effects do hard and soft water have on the shower spray heads?
2 Describe how hair condition and subsequent salon services are affected by the pH value of the products used.
3 What effect does an alkaline shampoo have on the hair?
4 Why is it sometimes useful to use an acid-balanced shampoo?
5 Describe the special types of shampoo that would be most suitable for the following:
   ■ greasy hair
   ■ scalps with dandruff
   ■ naturally dry hair
   ■ chemically dry hair
   ■ fine, flyaway hair
   ■ hair with excessive hairspray
   ■ hair about to be permed in the salon
   ■ afro-Caribbean hair?
6 Describe the massage movements used during shampooing, and name two occasions when scalp massage should *not* be used.
7 Would you expect to use more or less shampoo in a soft water area?
8 Why is it always important to follow the manufacturer's shampoo instructions?

Conditioning

A

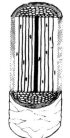

B

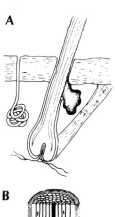

Test your knowledge

You will need to remember some facts about the hair and scalp to understand how conditioners work.

1 Scalp structure. Label each of the following on diagram A:
   ■ a sweat gland
   ■ a sebaceous gland
   ■ the dermis
   ■ the epidermis
   ■ a hair follicle
   ■ the blood supply
   ■ a hair.
2 Hair structure. Label the three main parts of the hair on diagram B.
3 Briefly describe the outer layer of the hair, including its colour.
4 Briefly describe the cortex in relation to hair condition.

Reasons for conditioning hair

Many clients complain 'I can't do a thing with my hair at the moment!'. Several things could be causing this:

Remember

Virgin hair is hair that has **never been chemically treated** but can still be in poor condition and need a conditioning treatment.

- **Physical and handling damage**, e.g. bad brushing and combing, over-drying the hair, excessive use of electrical treatments, excessive tension (elastic bands, tight ponytails), weathering (sunlight, sea and wind).
- **Chemical damage**, e.g. perming (over-processed perms), relaxing (over-processed hair straighteners), bleaching and highlighting (bleach left on too long), tinting (tint applied on top of tint), use of incompatible chemicals (hair-colour restorers and hydrogen peroxide). Look back at Chapter 1 for more details on how the hair can be damaged.
- **Medical history** (internal factors), e.g. poor health, poor diet (anorexia often causes hair loss), hormonal changes (pregnancy may cause hair loss and perm failure), courses of medication or drugs (people with cancer may lose their hair during treatment), stress.

You can help to restore the hair and scalp to a healthier state by offering the client a series of conditioning treatments which, combined with special scalp massages, will also help to relax the client.

Treating hair and scalp conditions

To do

Go back to Chapter 1 and re-read the sections on:

- hair structure
- scalp structure
- non-infectious hair and scalp conditions.

Hair conditions

Fragilitas crinium (split ends)
This is caused by harsh physical or chemical damage. The best treatment is to cut off the split ends.

On dry hair take a small, square section of the damaged hair and twist it. Rub the twisted strand of hair between your thumb and first finger so that the shorter, split ends stick out. These ends are easy to see as they are often white in colour. Hold the twisted hair firmly while you cut off the split ends.

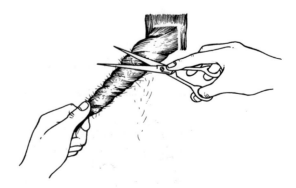

Re-conditioning treatments will also help split, damaged ends.

Damaged cuticle

The cuticle can be damaged by harsh physical and chemical treatment (remember the pH scale). Once the cuticle scales are raised and the hair feels rough, the hairs will easily matt together and tangle.

Conditioning treatments will help to smooth over and fill in the gaps between the cuticle scales, making the surface appear shiny again. Restructurants will also help to strengthen hair with damaged cuticle scales, as they are easily absorbed through the open scales.

Trichorrhexis nodosa

This is caused by harsh physical damage (elastic bands) or by chemical damage (perm rubbers fastened too tightly during perm processing).

If the hair can be cut then do so; if not (for example, if the breakage is near the roots) the hair will benefit from reconditioning or restructurants.

Scalp conditions

Pityriasis capitis (dandruff)

This is caused by overactive production of the skin cells on the scalp. It is noticeable as small, itchy, dry scales, white or grey in colour. Dandruff shampoos such as selenium sulphide (e.g. Selsun) and zinc pyrithione (e.g. Head and Shoulders) will lift the skin flakes off the scalp, but should not be used for long periods of time. A few weeks of use should suffice to get rid of the dandruff, then revert to a mild shampoo, using the dandruff shampoos only if the condition recurs.

Dry dandruff may also be treated with oil conditioners or special conditioning creams.

Seborrhoea (greasy hair and scalp)

This is caused by overactive sebaceous glands. It is often due to hormonal changes, and teenagers in particular may suffer from it. Seborrhoea can be controlled by shampoos for greasy hair or special spirit lotions.

Generally advise a client with this condition to avoid stimulating the sebaceous glands, i.e. not to brush the hair too much, not to rub the scalp too much during shampooing and not to use very hot water during shampooing.

To do

List the preparations used in your salon to treat the following conditions:

- fragilitas crinium
- damaged cuticle
- trichorrhexis nodosa
- pityriasis capitis
- seborrhoea.

Types of conditioner

Oil conditioners

Olive oil, almond oil and coconut oil are pure vegetable oils which can be applied to dry hair then processed with heat. They will make the hair feel soft, supple and shiny.

Acid rinses

Weak acids (pH 4–5), such as lemon juice and vinegar (mix 1 tablespoon to 1 pint warm water) can be poured through the hair after shampooing and left on. They will make the hair shiny by closing the cuticle scales.

Chemicals, such as neutralisers, bleaches and permanent tints are alkaline (opening the cuticle scales) and work by adding oxygen to the hair. To return the hair to its natural (acid) state we need to use **ascorbic acid**. This **antioxidant** (i.e. it removes oxygen) is often added to acid-balanced conditioners because of its antioxidant properties, and because it closes the cuticles.

Leave-in conditioners

These contain **moisturising and protective** ingredients and are sprayed on to wet hair, making it easier to comb. They are ideal for greasy, **fine or tight curly afro hair** and are very useful for **disentangling children's hair**. They also prevent the hair from drying too quickly during cutting.

Conditioning creams (surface conditioners)

Ordinary conditioning creams are emulsions, which work in a similar way to the hair's natural grease (sebum). They coat the hair with a thin film, filling in some of the gaps in the broken cuticle scales so the hair becomes more shiny and manageable. They are applied after shampooing and rinsed out of the hair. The better ones are acid balanced.

Deep-acting conditioners

These are sometimes used when reconditioning the hair, especially as a part of a 4–6 week series of weekly treatments for hair in very poor condition.

They are usually thicker than ordinary conditioning creams, and stick to the hair better after rinsing (they are **substantive** to the hair). This is because they are cationic – they have a positive electrical charge, which makes them stick to the hair shaft and remain there.

Restructurants

Hair that is in a very weakened and over-processed (over-permed or over-bleached) state, such as in trichorrhexis nodosa, will benefit from the application of a restructurant. Restructurants should be applied to shampooed, towel-dried hair and left on (not rinsed off).

Restructurants often contain protein hydrolysates and are sometimes known as **protein** conditioners (or **penetrating** conditioners). They help to strengthen the hair and can be used before chemical treatments as for a series of reconditioning treatments.

When to apply conditioners for chemical processes

Before chemical processing – protective conditioner

Hair that is in poor condition may need either a special type of restructurant, or, in the case of perming, a pre-perm conditioner.

Damaged hair is often more porous and will absorb perm lotion very quickly. Some hair is unevenly porous in places, for example on the ends, and may need a pre-perm lotion applied specifically to those areas to even out the porosity.

After chemical processing – corrective conditioner

Acid-balanced conditioning creams are particularly good after perming, bleaching and tinting because they help to replace lost moisture, close down the cuticle scales and work as antioxidants.

Application of conditioners

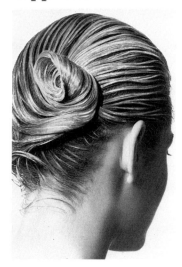

- Decide whether you are treating the **hair** or the **scalp** condition. If it is the hair, then apply the conditioner to the hair. If it is the scalp, apply the conditioner to the scalp.
- Check whether the product needs to be applied to **dry** or to **wet** hair. Oils (e.g. olive oil) are applied to dry hair.
- If the product is to be applied to wet hair after shampooing, always towel dry the hair, or the product will be diluted.
- Always **disentangle the hair** and apply the conditioner according to the manufacturer's directions. Section the hair and apply with a brush as you would apply a tint.
- Use a rake comb (a wide-toothed comb) to comb the product through the hair, to distribute it evenly along the length of the hair. NB: products used for scalp treatments (e.g. dandruff, seborrhoea) do not need to be combed through the hair.
- Check the manufacturer's processing times. When processing is complete, rinse the product from the hair. Remember that oil conditioners need to be shampooed out.

To do
■ Check all the conditioning products in your salon and read the instructions to see how they are applied and how long they should be left on the hair.

Scalp massage

Scalp massage is done once the conditioner has been applied. It is very **relaxing** and should be done in a calm atmosphere.

During massage the scalp reddens (this is called **hyperaemia**) because the blood supply to the skin surface is increased. When this happens more blood comes to the base of the hair follicle, encouraging hair growth. Have you noticed how your skin becomes red in the summer when the weather is hot or when you have been exercising? When this happens the blood is coming to the skin surface to cool you down, but it is also feeding your hair follicles. That is why your hair (and nails) grow more quickly in the summer and why your client's hair will be encouraged to grow when you give a hand scalp massage.

Contra-indications

Never massage the scalp:

- when there are any **infections** (e.g. ringworm) or infestations (e.g. head lice) present
- if there are any **cuts or abrasions** on the scalp
- if the scalp is **inflamed** or sore to touch
- if the client has any **medical problems**, even a high temperature, as with colds or 'flu.

Massage movements

Effleurage

This is a **stroking movement,** which begins and ends the massage procedure. With your fingers spread slightly apart and starting at the front hairline, apply an even pressure as you slowly slide your fingers through the hair down to the nape in a continuous movement. You should cover most parts of the scalp with your fingers, so that when you repeat the movement several times the client starts to relax.

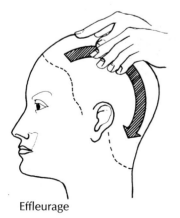

Effleurage

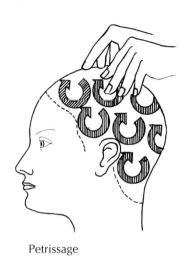

Petrissage

Petrissage

This is a **deeper, kneading movement**, using the pads of the fingers. It stimulates the muscles and nerves, improving the blood circulation. Move your finger pads in a circular direction, picking up and kneading the scalp.

People with a lot of thick hair often have a 'mobile' scalp which is easy to knead, but others with fine, thin hair may have a tight scalp which is more difficult to work with. Take care not to pull fine, sparse hair.

Always ask the client if your massage is comfortable. If you are unsure about the amount of pressure to use, try out the massage on your own scalp first.

During petrissage, start at the front hairline, knead around the top of the head, then gradually work towards the nape area. This massage may last for 5–10 minutes.

Friction

This is a **light, rubbing movement** using the finger pads. It is stimulating rather than relaxing and it is not always carried out. It is only done for a few minutes, again working from front to back.

Using heat to assist the penetration of conditioners

Applying heat to oils, conditioning creams, and deep-acting conditioners will encourage them to penetrate further into the hair.

Steamers

These look like hand hairdryers but must be warmed up before use. They produce **moist heat** through the evaporation of distilled water (tap water would make them fur up – like a kettle). The steam swells the hair and raises the cuticle scales so that the product can penetrate more thoroughly. Steamers are particularly useful for Afro hair.

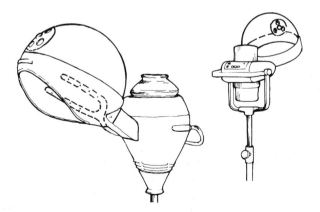

Steamers

Accelerators

These use an infra-red light to produce **dry heat**, which helps penetration. A plastic cap may need to be used to stop the product from drying out.

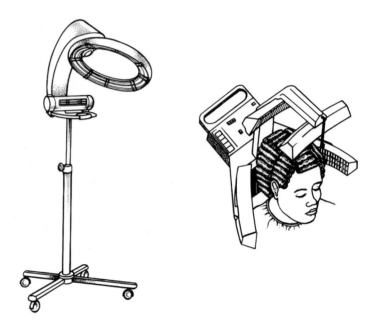

Accelerators

Hood dryers

These also produce a **dry heat**. Hot, dry air circulates to dry the hair. A plastic cap is placed over the hair and product before use. Remember to warm the hood dryer first by turning it on for several minutes before the client is ready to use it.

Record cards

Always keep record cards of the client's treatments. Here is an example:

TREATMENT RECORD CARD

Name

Address

Tel. no.

Date	Hair condition	Scalp condition	Product used	Equipment used	Time	Other details	Stylist

The client could have both hair problems (e.g. over-processed, dry ends) and scalp problems (e.g. a naturally greasy scalp) at the same time. If this is the case, deal with the worst problem first, then, when this has been corrected, start to treat the second problem.

Test your knowledge

1 Briefly describe how the structure of hair relates to conditioning treatments.
2 What is the name of the gland which can cause seborrhoea?
3 Which part of the scalp causes pityriasis capitis?
4 Why is it sometimes beneficial to apply conditioners before chemical processing and at other times after chemical processing?
5 What is the name of the substance that conditions hair naturally?
6 Name the differences between each massage technique.
7 Describe the benefits of scalp massage.
8 State when scalp massage should not be used.
9 Describe why the pH of various products is important to both hair condition and subsequent salon services.

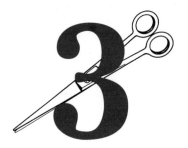

Blow drying

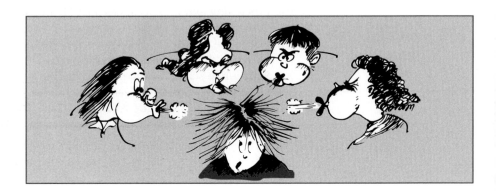

Hair types and textures

You will need to understand the different hair types (European, Negroid or Asian) and textures (fine or coarse) to know what **tools** (e.g. size of brush), **techniques** (e.g. blow dry, scrunch dry) and **products** (e.g. blow dry lotion, mousse or gel) to use.

Hair growth patterns

To do

■ Re-read the section in Chapter 1 on hair growth patterns.

Natural growth patterns and root movement are just as important when blow drying as when cutting. If you blow dry **with the natural fall** (the way the hair falls on its own) the style will last longer and the client will find it easier to manage.

To do

■ Re-read the section in Chapter 1 on designing a hairstyle to suit your client.

Why the shape of hair can change through blow drying

All hair is elastic and stretchy. It becomes more elastic when it is thoroughly wet, when it can stretch up to half its length again.

Wet hair stretches because the **temporary bonds** (the hydrogen bonds and salt links) that join the polypeptide chains in the cortex **are broken**. However, they quickly rejoin into a new shape when you blow dry the hair.

You can blow dry:

and

curly and wavy hair ⟶ straight

straight hair ⟶ wavy

by breaking the temporary bonds, stretching the hair with a brush and then drying it.

Hair in its natural state – whether curly, wavy or straight – is described as being in an **alpha keratin** state. When the hair is wetted, stretched into a new shape and then dried, it is in a **beta keratin** state.

Once the hair is dampened again – by shampooing or just by being caught out in the rain – then it will go back to its natural state (curly, wavy or straight) and be in the alpha keratin state again.

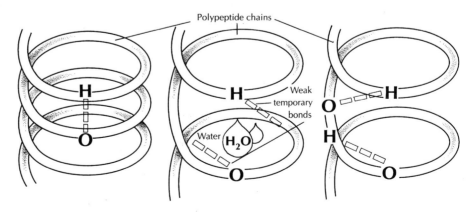

ALPHA KERATIN
Dry hair unstretched

BETA KERATIN
Wet hair stretched

BETA KERATIN
Stretched position

Blow-drying aids and products

Your hair goes flat when the weather is damp and miserable because hair is **hygroscopic**. This means it **absorbs moisture from the atmosphere** and the stretched (beta keratin) blow-dried shape reverts to its natural (alpha keratin) shape.

To stop this from happening, and to make the blow dry last longer, we use blow-dry lotion, mousse or gel. These work in the same way as hairspray, in that they **coat the hair with a very fine film of plastic** to stop the hair absorbing moisture.

It is important to use products intended for blow drying – setting lotions will make the hair too sticky to work with.

Always apply blow-dry aids to towel-dried hair, because if the hair is too wet the product will be diluted. Check the manufacturer's instructions, but you will find that you should apply most gels and mousses by placing them in the centre of your palm and then spreading them evenly over the hair with your fingers. Blow dry lotions must be sprinkled evenly over the hair.

To do

■ The client will have already been gowned up for shampooing. Check with your supervisor if a special colour towel is needed whilst applying colour products, which could stain light-coloured towels.

Remember

The COSHH Act (see Chapter 10)
You are responsible. Hairspray and many other hairdressing products are highly flammable, so do not store them in direct sunlight or use them if clients are smoking.
Don't spray aerosols onto the client's skin or into their eyes – and use them in well ventilated areas wherever possible.

Some blow-dry products contain colours, such as silver, ash or copper, which wash out of the hair. Only use these with the help of your supervisor or once you have learned about colouring (this is described in Chapter 6) – you may find the hair turns out the colour of a carrot!

To do

Find out which blow dry products in your salon are suitable for:

■ fine hair
■ coarse hair
■ curly hair
■ straight hair
■ a soft or casual look
■ a firm hold
■ a wild, full look.

Finally, after blow drying you can use a hairspray for extra hold, or spray-on shine or wax for a glossy finish.

Tools and equipment

Brushes

Flat brushes

These are good for smooth finishes, especially for bob haircuts. They are not recommended for very curly results.

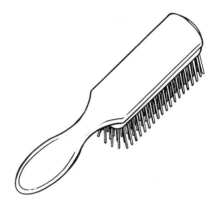

Vent brushes

These have open spaces at the back to allow air flow during blow drying. They are quick and easy to use, but can become tangled in the hair. They are good for breaking up the style to produce a soft, casual effect.

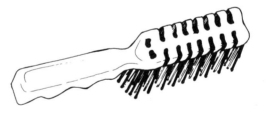

Circular brushes

These come in a variety of sizes and are useful for producing a curled effect. The smaller the brush, the smaller the finished curl.

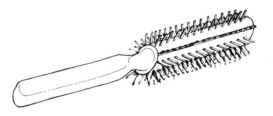

Combs

Rake combs

These combs are used for disentangling the hair after shampooing. They always have widely spaced teeth, and do not tear or stretch wet hair.

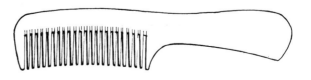

Cutting salon combs (straight combs)

These have two sizes of teeth and are made in various lengths and sizes. The longer teeth are useful for disentangling hair.

Use this type of comb for sectioning the hair before blow drying and while assessing the natural growth patterns and root lift.

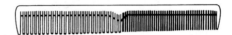

Sectioning clips

Sectioning clips or butterfly clamps are needed to hold large sections of hair apart during blow drying.

Electrical appliances

Hand hairdryers

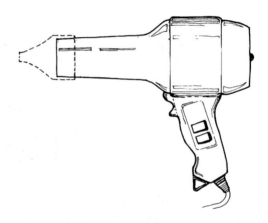

Precautions
- Make sure all plugs are wired correctly.
- Always check the heat setting and speed controls **before** you start blow drying.
- Make sure that the dryer cable and plug are always safe (look out for frayed wires and loose plug tops).
- Hairdryers have an air intake grill at the back, which must be cleaned regularly to remove dust and fluff. If they are not cleaned regularly they may overheat and become dangerous.

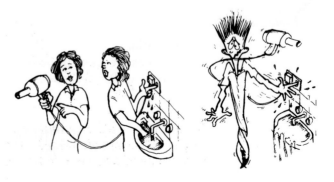

HEALTH MATTERS

Standing all day long

Arms and body

Muscles are used for two kinds of work, dynamic and static. **Dynamic work** is when the muscles are moving and the blood is pumping through them. **Static work** is when the muscles are being held in position. This can restrict the blood flow, causing waste products to accumulate and making the muscles tired, tense and stiff. Therefore, you should keep your muscles as relaxed as possible by changing the way in which you hold yourself.

For instance, move around your client when you are working on the sides of their hair – don't stand at the back and stretch over or you could strain your back.

It is also useful to learn how to use the hairdryer and brush with either hand, swapping over occasionally. This will help to keep the weight of the dryer balanced by using both arms. Sometimes the lead of the dryer will not reach around the client, so you **have** to use both hands!

Attachments

Nozzles

When these are attached to the hairdryer the **airflow is concentrated**, which is useful for drying small sections of hair.

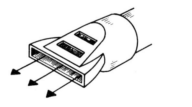 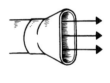

Diffusers

These have the opposite effect to a nozzle. With a diffuser, the air is **dispersed over a wider area** and the airflow is less forceful. They are often used for drying permed hair.

Electric tongs

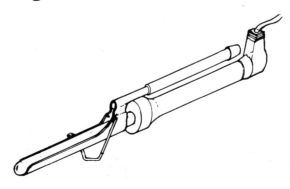

Tongs can be used to produce a variety of effects, from curls and waves to ringlets. They are often used after blow drying to **'firm up' the shape of the curl** produced by a circular brush.

The ends of the hair must be smoothly wound around the tongs – or else you will produce distorted or buckled ends.

All tongs have a thermostat inside them to prevent overheating but remember that they can still burn. Many also have a flex with a swivel action to prevent the cord from becoming twisted.

To do

Health and safety requirements
■ Read the Electricity at Work Regulations 1990 and the section on using electrical equipment safely in Chapter 10.
■ Make a list of any pieces of electrical equipment in your salon that you think are unsafe. Check it with your supervisor.

Hot brushes

Hot brushes are easier to use than tongs but you cannot achieve quite as many different effects (such as ringlets) with them. Again, they have a thermostat inside them and the flex may have a swivel action.

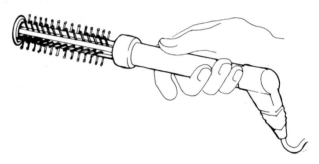

Hot brushes work in the same way as tongs but the teeth or bristles help to grip the hair. They can be easier to work with than tongs, but you must take **clean sections** or they can become tangled in the hair.

Crimping irons

These are used on straight hair to produce a pattern of **straight-line crimps** in the hair. They create volume, making the hair appear thicker, and are useful for long hair.

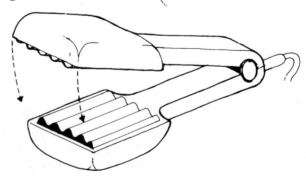

Remember

Tongs, hot brushes and crimping irons should be cleaned with cotton wool or disinfectant spray or wipes – **never** immersed in water.

To use the crimpers, take neat sections of the hair no wider than the metal plates of the crimpers and close the iron for 2–5 seconds on the hair. Release, then move down to the next part of the straight hair, press again and release. Continue until all the hair is crimped.

Precautions for using tongs, hot brushes and crimping irons

- Always pick them up by their **handles**.
- Always place a **comb** between hot tongs and the client's scalp when you are working near the scalp.

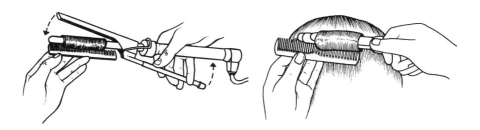

- Always use the **stand or rest** attached to the tongs to prevent work surfaces from becoming scorched, and plastic surfaces (such as equipment trolleys) from becoming melted.
- Never put hot tongs into your tool bag. Allow them to **cool** first.
- Remember to **switch off** the tongs as soon as you have finished using them – it helps to prevent accidents.
- Light-coloured hair can be discoloured and scorched by the tongs, so do not have them **too hot** or use them for **too long** on the hair.
- All flexes can become twisted and the insulation can gradually wear away, making the tools dangerous. Flexes must be **checked regularly**.

Using mirrors when blow drying

During blow drying, as with combing out and finishing the style, you need to look continually in the mirror to check the balance of the hairstyle. You must make sure it is not lop-sided or that there are any large breaks or holes in the dressing.

Technical points to remember when blow drying

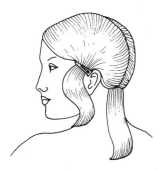

Hair sectioned for blow drying

- Always **towel dry** the hair first (except for very curly, very fine or very short hair) to save drying time, then use any blow drying aids.
- A style always lasts longer if it follows the **natural fall**.
- Comb the hair in the direction of the finished style, then **section** according to the size of the brush you have chosen. Ensure that dry sections do not mix with wet sections.
- Make sure each section is **thoroughly dry** before you take the next section.

Blow-drying techniques

Drying method	Effect	Suitability
Flat brush	Used for a smooth finish, e.g. a 'bob'	Hair requiring only a slight curve or straight finish; curl cannot be achieved
Vent brush	Produces a soft, casual, 'broken up' effect	Good for a quick casual result, but not very suitable for curling
Circular brush	Good for producing a curled effect; the smaller the brush the tighter the finished curl	Large circular brushes are used to curl the ends of long hair. Small brushes give tight curls. Any circular brush tangles easily in the hair
Finger drying	Produces a very natural, soft look	Best used for 'fashion' looks. If the client bends forwards and the hair is dried from underneath more lift is achieved at the roots
Natural drying (diffuser, accelerator, infra-red, roller ball)	Produces a natural look similar to the shape of the hair when wet	Ideal for drying permed or naturally curly hair, as the hair is not disturbed when drying
Scrunch drying	Produces a rough finish with lots of movement	Works best on medium-length, layered hair with some wave and movement

- The **root area** is normally dried first – to increase volume the outflow should be directed towards the roots.

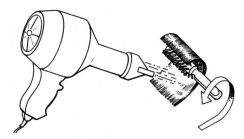

Drying into roots to increase volume

- Always **work from roots to points**, keeping the cuticle scale flat.

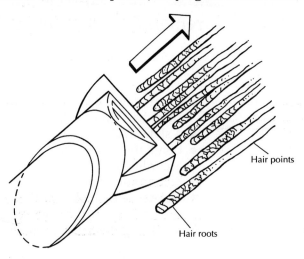

Hair points

Hair roots

Keeping the cuticle scale flat

- Keep the dryer **moving** to prevent burning the hair or the scalp.
- Always **lift the hair** whilst removing the brush to prevent tangling.
- Keep an **even tension** on the hair but do not overstretch it by pulling too hard.

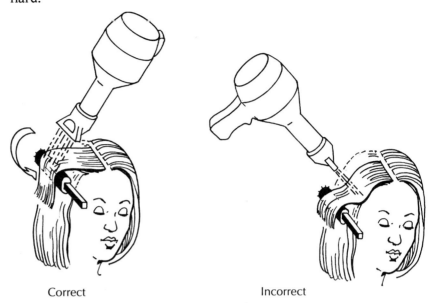

Correct   Incorrect

- Allow hair to **cool completely** (cold shots of air from the dryer help), then check it is quite dry. Warm hair can be deceptively damp.
- Keep **checking the shape** of the hairstyle in the mirror, and always show your client the back.

HEALTH MATTERS

Styling

It is as important when styling to work at the correct height of the client (by adjusting the chair height or by bending your knees) as it is when cutting.

Are your shoes comfortable? Shoes that pinch and are too tight will increase strain, and ones with heels that are too high will cause undue back stress and may make you too tall for the client's height in the chair.

Try to take little breaks when working to rest your arms and hands. This is easily done by stopping to explain to your client how to maintain their style or which products (shampoos, conditioners, styling products or hairsprays) they could use at home.

Finishing products

Hairsprays

These are used to **hold the style** and often contain ingredients to enhance the shine. They must be **sprayed 30 cm away** from the hair – too close and they will clog the hair and cause a build-up.

Gels and waxes

These give the strongest hold and shine. They are used for **controlling frizz and static**, **defining** the line, **slicking** hair back and **moulding and sculpting**.

Pomades and dressing creams

These have the **same uses as gels and waxes** but are gentler on the hair.

Moisturisers, serums and activators

These oil sprays are also known as leave-in conditioners but may be used on dry hair to **reduce static** and aid **gloss or shine**. They must be used **sparingly** by spray misting over the hair or by applying them to the palms of the hands, rubbing the hands together and then smoothing on the hair.

To do

- Find out the names of all the finishing products used in your salon.
- Look out four different pictures of hairstyles and decide which is the best finishing product for each one. Check the answers with your supervisor.

Test your knowledge

1 Make a list of three different textures and types of hair.
2 Why do you have to consider hair growth patterns when blow drying?
3 State two differences between the properties of wet and dry hair.
4 Describe the effects of humidity on dried hair.
5 Name three different blow-drying effects.
6 Describe the tools, equipment and products you would use to achieve these effects.
7 Which government act relates to the use of electrical drying equipment? Briefly describe its contents.
8 Name the government act that relates to finishing products. Describe how these products may be hazardous.

Afro hair

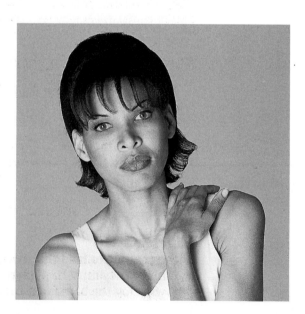

Temporarily straightened Afro hair

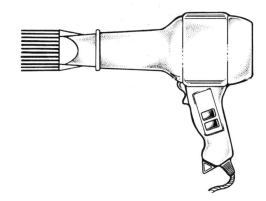

Afro hair does not blow dry well unless it has been temporarily straightened by **soft pressing** or by using a wide-toothed comb hand dryer attachment. Once the hair is straight it can be moulded into shape with the dryer and circular brushes.

Pressing combs

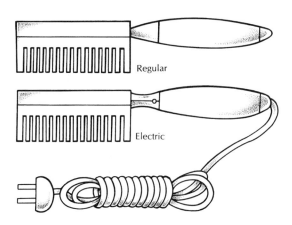

Regular

Electric

Regular or non-electric combs

These combs are made of steel or brass and the handle is made of wood. They are heated by small electric heaters or gas stoves. Eight sizes are available, the space between the teeth varying – small teeth are used for fine hair, large teeth for coarse hair.

Thermostatically controlled combs

These have a set working temperature.

Soft pressing

Always **check the scalp for soreness** (from chemical treatments) or **scratches** (from previous pressing or styling) before proceeding. **Do not continue** if this is the case, but recommend conditioning treatments.

Using this method 70% of the curl can be removed.

The technique

- **Shampoo**, **condition** and **dry** the hair.
- Apply a suitable **pressing oil**, **pomade** or **cream** to the **hair and scalp** to protect against scorching and add sheen.

- Take **sections** of **1.25 cm**, starting at the back and holding the hair at **90° to the head**. Check the heat of the comb, then insert it **1.25 cm from the scalp**.

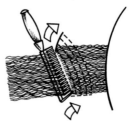

Inserting a pressing comb

- Slide the comb down the hair mesh, turning it over so that the **back of the comb** creates tension and straightens the hair.

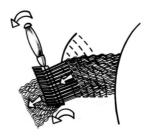

Pulling hair straight using back of pressing comb

- **Comb each mesh** of hair **two or three times** and gradually work towards the front.
- Once **complete**, apply a dressing cream, brush it through and **style** with curling tongs.

Hard pressing

This method removes almost all of the curl but is more damaging to the hair than soft pressing. Simply **repeat the soft pressing** method or **straighten the hair again** with **marcel waving irons**. These non-electric irons are slid down the hair mesh, pulling it straight.

Cleaning pressing combs

Always wipe the pressing comb free from grease and loose hairs after use. **Clean combs work better**, so use a commercially prepared product regularly to help remove carbon build-up.

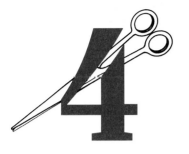

Cutting

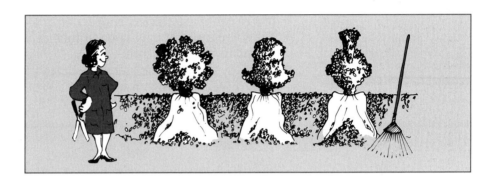

More clients visit the hairdresser for cutting than for any other service, because it is impossible for an untrained person to achieve as good a cut. A good haircut is the basis of every hairstyle and can completely change a client's view of themselves.

The hairdresser can remove both length and thickness by cutting, and create a completely new shape or style.

Gowning up

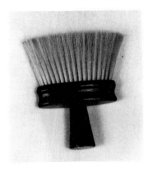

There is nothing more irritating for a client than leaving the salon covered in pieces of hair. Hairs not only fall down the back of clothing, but get stuck in all sorts of fabrics and clothes (especially sweaters) and are difficult to remove. So gown up properly.

Gowns are used to cover the client's clothes, and shoulder capes can be used around the client's shoulders. Clean towels may be placed around the client's neck during wet cutting but, as cut hairs embed themselves into towels, it is more hygienic to towel-dry the hair and use cutting collars for protection.

To prevent cut hairs from falling into the client's clothing, insert a strip of **cotton wool** or **neck tissue** around the neck area. These are disposable and should be used only once.

Wet-cut hairs are especially difficult to remove from the skin, but the use of **talcum powder** and a **neck brush** makes their removal easier.

Always keep a clothes' brush at reception to remove hairs from the client's clothes after the gown and cape are removed.

| To do |

■ Re-read the section on designing a hairstyle to suit your client in Chapter 1.

Advantages of cutting hair dry

Remember

Wet hair stretches much more than dry hair and when it dries it can become **very much shorter**.

- Hair is **not as elastic** or stretchy as when wet, so you can see the true length as you cut.
- You **can see split ends** clearly to cut them off (see Chapter 2).
- It is easier to use **electric clippers** on dry hair.
- The client may not have **enough time or money** for a wet cut, but be willing to have a dry trim.
- If you are thinning the haircut with special thinning scissors you will remove less hair when it is dry.

Advantages of cutting hair wet

- The hair is **clean** and **not as tangled** as it is when dry (easier to comb).
- You can see the **natural fall** clearly only when the hair is wet.
- **Precision cutting** is always done on wet hair because cutting guidelines can be seen clearly.
- **More varied cutting techniques,** e.g. razor cutting and slide cutting, can be used on wet hair.

Hair thickness and waviness

Fine and coarse hair

See Chapter 1 regarding the different thicknesses of hair. Very thin or **fine hair** can be difficult to cut because, unless you are careful, 'steps' can appear.

On the other hand, some hair is so coarse and wiry that only very sharp tools (scissors and razors), used on fine sub-sections, will cut it easily.

Curly and straight hair

There are three main racial hair types:

- **European** – generally wavy
- **Asian** (including Chinese and Japanese hair) – usually straight
- **Negroid** or Afro-Caribbean – very curly.

All need to be cut differently.

Generally, **straight hair** must be cut carefully or 'steps' will appear, and more movement can be produced by layering and thinning.

People with **curly hair** will find that if their long hair is cut short it will appear even curlier! This is because the weight of long hair stretches it and it appears more wavy than curly.

The natural fall of hair

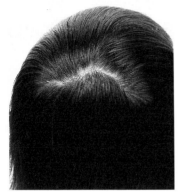

Double crown

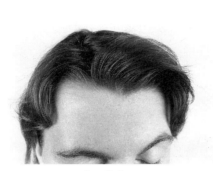

Cowlick

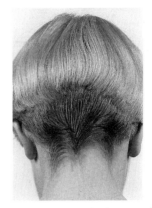

Nape whorl

To do

Re-read the section in Chapter 2 on hair growth patterns, noting how to cut hair with:

- a double crown
- a cowlick
- a nape whorl
- a widow's peak.

Test your knowledge

1 State how the following critical factors can influence your choice of haircut:
   - hair structure
   - hair texture
   - head and face shape
   - hair growth patterns.
2 Give examples of how you would advise your client to select a suitable style.

Cutting tools

All cutting tools must be **sharp**, in **good condition**, **clean** and **sterile**, and should **never** be **kept in pockets** or left around out of their case.

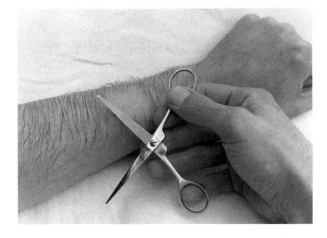

These are the most commonly used tools in cutting.

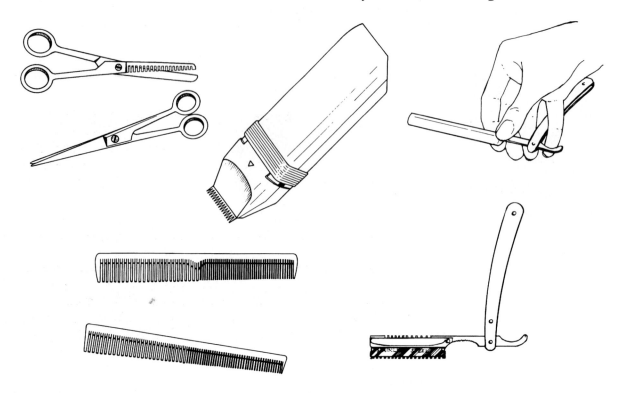

Scissors

Good-quality scissors are made of well-tempered or cobalt steel and are available in various sizes – from 10 cm to 18 cm from the tip of the blade to the handles. Many hairdressers prefer to use short scissors for precision cutting, but long scissors are useful for other techniques such as those used for cutting Afro-Caribbean hair and barbering.

Looking after your scissors

- **Never** use them for cutting anything **other than hair** – they will quickly become blunt.
- **Always** keep the **blades dry** by wiping them with cotton wool and surgical spirit (this will also disinfect the blades).
- Lightly **oil** the blades and the pivot screw if they start to feel stiff and awkward to use.

> **Remember**
>
> Scissors are very expensive. Look after them properly.

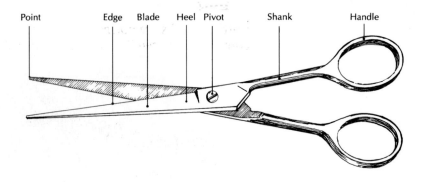

- **Try not to drop your scissors** – the blades may be damaged and the pivot screw (which balances the scissors) could work loose.
- Keep your scissors in their original **protective case** for safety and to prevent them being damaged.
- If your scissors need mending or sharpening, always send them to a **professional hairdressing scissors company** (advertisements are found in hairdressing trade journals).

HEALTH MATTERS

Choose your scissors carefully – they must fit the size of your hand and feel comfortable to work with. Try asking different stylists in your salon if you may hold their scissors to see how they feel.

During cutting keep your wrist in a straight line from middle finger to elbow, to prevent wrist strain. Before starting a haircut always adjust the height of your chair or bend from your knees, keeping your back straight to make sure you are not bending incorrectly. Face forwards and look down slightly. If your head is slanted too much it means that its weight is being supported by your neck muscles instead of your bones and can result in strain, neck pain or headaches. A cutting stool is an excellent idea as it allows you to work at the correct height and can be moved from side to side around the client.

Holding your scissors

You can always spot a professional hairdresser by the way they pick up and hold a pair of scissors using their thumb and **third** finger. They do this to achieve maximum control during cutting.

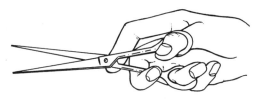

To do

- Practise holding your scissors and opening and closing the blades. One blade is kept still whilst the other is opened and closed with your thumb.
- Now try this movement again, rotating your wrist at the same time.

Combs

Cutting combs are normally used during cutting, but fine flexible barber's combs can be used if you need to cut really short neck hairs.

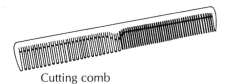

Cutting comb

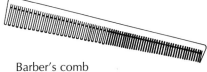

Barber's comb

During cutting the sub-section of hair to be cut is held in the fingers of one hand and the scissors in the other. To hold the comb at the same time, palm the scissors for safety and hold the comb in your scissors hand.

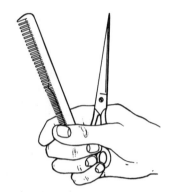

Palming the scissors

To do

■ Practise taking your thumb out of the scissor handles, closing the scissors and holding the comb at the same time.

Cutting techniques using scissors

Club cutting

This is the most common cutting technique. However, it must be precise and is often called **precision** cutting.

The sub-section of hair must be cleanly combed through and held with an even tension before cutting.

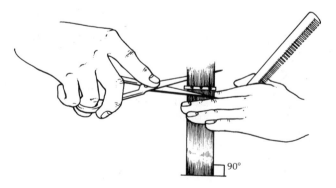

The diagram shows hair cut at 90° for a layer cut, but the hair may be cut at any angle to the head according to the style planned. Club cutting may be done on wet or dry hair and the ends of the hair are left blunt and heavy (this is sometimes also called **blunt** cutting).

Taper cutting

Taper, **slither** or **feather** cutting will reduce both the length and the thickness of the hair. This technique is done on dry hair and, unlike club cutting (where the hair is cut over the fingers), the hair is cut underneath the fingers.

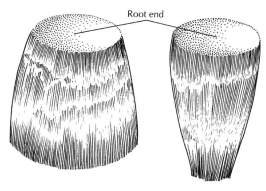

Root end

Club cut hair   Taper cut hair

Tapering is a sliding, slithering, backwards-and-forwards movement along a sub-section of hair. Close the scissor blades as you move towards the roots.

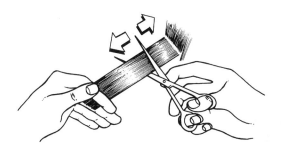

Remember

All these techniques will give lots of variations of cuts, but it is the angle at which you hold the hair that gives the greatest differences in style.

To do

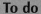

- Practise the action of taper cutting by opening and closing your scissors in slow motion, at the same time moving the points of the scissors away from you then back towards you.

Pointing and texturing

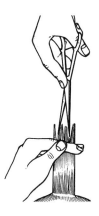

Pointing can be used to achieve feathered effects and to soften hard lines created by club cutting.

Take a sub-section of hair and insert the scissors over the fingers to chip out small pieces at the ends of the hair.

When larger pieces are taken out of the hair this is called **texturising**.

Scissor over comb

This technique is used to give the **same effect as clipper over comb work** – the hair around the nape and sides is cut short, following the contours of the head.

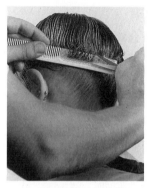

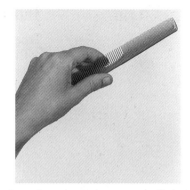

Use a cutting comb to pick up the hair, keeping the scissors parallel to the comb during cutting. Use the comb in an upwards direction, lifting the hair so that the hair sticking through it can be cut off. Move the comb and scissors continually towards the top of the head, keeping the comb up and out and away from the head, cutting at the same time.

Thinning hair with thinning scissors

These scissors remove only **thickness** or bulk from the hair, **not length**. They are sometimes called **aesculaps**, **serrated** or **texturising** scissors.

Ordinary thinning scissors can be used to thin out from the middle of the hair, cutting diagonally across the sub-section of the hair. Open and close them two or three times to remove the thickness.

Remember
Use thinning scissors only on **dry hair** – you could thin the hair too much if the hair is wet.
Do not thin:
■ around the hairline
■ at the crown area
■ too close to the scalp
■ along any partings
because spiky ends will result.

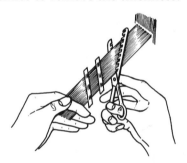

Many new variations on the normal thinning scissors, with different shapes of blades to create lots of exciting effects, have been developed.

Cutting techniques using clippers and razors

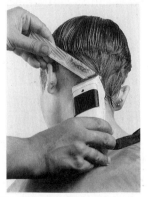

Clipper over comb technique

Clippers

Electric clippers are now commonly used for both men's and women's hairdressing to give the same effect as the 'scissor over comb' technique. They have two blades with sharp-edged teeth. One blade remains fixed while the other moves across it. The action of the motorised moving blade is similar to several pairs of scissors being used at the same time, which is why many hairdressers like the speed of cutting with clippers.

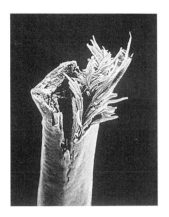

A hair cut with a blunt razor

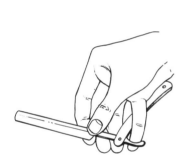

Open razor hold

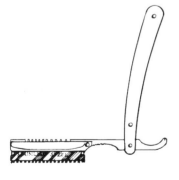

Safety razor

Detachable clipper heads are available so that the closeness of the cut can be altered. The **larger** the number, the **longer** the length; the **smaller** the number, the **shorter** the length.

Razors

Two main types of razor are in use:

- an **open** or **cut-throat** razor
- a **shaper** or **safety** razor.

Both are used on wet hair because razoring on dry hair is painful for the client. Razors must be kept sharp or they will tear the hair.

Open or cut-throat razors
Open razors may be used to **shorten** the hair and to **remove thickness**. They are used underneath or above the wet sub-sections of hair and are stroked towards the ends with a scooping movement that produces a tapered effect. Many hairdressers also use open razors to create a clean hairline around the haircut.

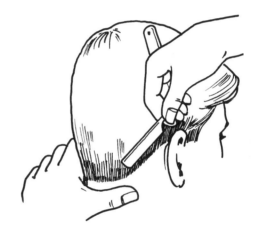

Hairline shaping

It is important to **hold a razor safely** so that it does not close up on your hand during cutting.

Open razors are now available with **disposable blades**. These are more hygienic, and as one blade becomes blunt you can replace it so you always have a sharp edge to use.

Shapers or safety razors
These razors have a guard over the blade so that only part of the hair is cut. They produce a **feathered**, **uneven** effect and are easier and safer to use than an open razor.

To do

The Health and Safety at Work Act 1974 requires you to **work safely**. Find the address of your local Health and Safety Executive (HSE) from your library or town hall and check the local bylaws regarding the use of razors.

Cutting tools and techniques

Technique	Tools	Cut wet or dry	Effects
Club cutting	Scissors Clippers	Wet or dry Dry	Removes length Hair curls less. Ends of hair look thicker
Taper cutting	Scissors Razor	Dry Wet	Removes length Removes thickness Hair curls more
Pointing and texturising	Scissors	Wet or dry	Removes thickness from the ends of the hair and can create a spiky, textured effect. Use to remove 'steps' in haircut
Scissor/clipper over comb	Scissors Clippers	Dry Dry	Removes length Used for short, often graduated haircuts
Thinning	Thinning scissors Razor	Dry Wet	Removes thickness from the hair

Points to remember during cutting

- You must have checked in your mind that the style will **suit** the client, but also make sure that you and the client are talking about the **same hairstyle**. Use a photograph if necessary.
- Check the **natural growths** (crown area, natural partings, etc.) again. Try to work **with** the hair, not against it – the client has to manage the style at home without your help.
- Use **section clips** to keep large sections of hair apart so that you can work cleanly.

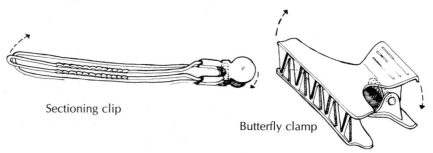

Sectioning clip

Butterfly clamp

- Keep your **cutting sections** small and narrow so that you can always see your guideline.
- Use an **open-tufted brush** (a vent brush) during cutting to brush the hair in different directions so you can see how well the hair is falling into shape.

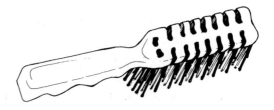

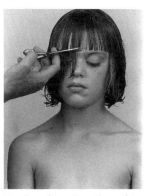

Freehand cutting (for a fringe with a cowlick)

- Always keep a **water spray** close at hand to dampen the hair if it starts to dry.
- Use the **mirrors** around the salon to check the shape of the client's haircut from various angles.
- **Hand mirrors** can also be used to check short graduations or bobs by placing them directly underneath the hairline.
- Do not pull the hair or use **too much tension** around the ears or when cutting a fringe over a cowlick – it may bounce up too short. Use freehand cutting instead.
- Check your client's **head position** – is it level? If their legs are crossed, then their head will be lop-sided – and so will your haircut!
- To make sure that the sides are level take **small strands** of hair from either side and gradually slide your fingers to the ends. If the strands have been taken from exactly the same place at each side your thumbs will be level.
- Use parts of the face (nose and eyes) to **check lengths** are equal.
- Ask the client throughout the cutting 'is this the **correct length**?'

Cutting tight curly Afro hair

<table>
<tr><td>Remember</td></tr>
<tr><td>Wet tight curly hair will spring back and become much shorter than expected, which is why it is better to cut it dry.</td></tr>
</table>

Afro hair that has been permed or straightened needs the same cutting techniques as straight, wavy or curly hair. However, naturally tight curly Afro hair needs different considerations.

- Always cut it **dry**, after shampooing and natural drying to achieve a perfect shape.
- Use a **wide-toothed afro comb** to lift it out from the head and remove any tangles.

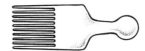

- Spray the hair lightly with a thin film of oil from an **instant moisturising spray** to make it easier to comb through.
- Use **freehand cutting** – do not hold the hair with your fingers. Allow the hair to fall naturally, then cut with scissors or clippers.
- Keep **lifting the hair** with the afro comb to check the shape and balance of the style.

Cutting angles and lines for different styles

There are only three style plans, from which all other styles can be achieved:

- the one-length cut
- the layer cut
- the graduation (layers graduating from long to short).

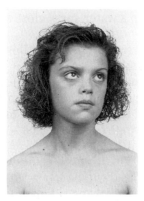

One-length cut

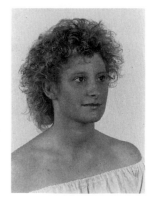

Layer cut

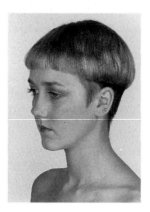

Short graduation

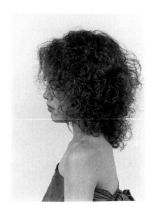

Long graduation

The one-length cut

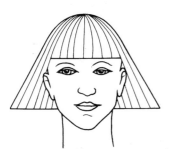

This is where the hair is cut to fall at the same outside length. Hair often looks **thicker** when cut in this style.

The guidelines are taken either horizontally or diagonally, starting at the hairline, and each section is taken parallel to the cutting line.

Always cut a one-length cut from the **natural fall**, from both the parting and the crown area, combing the hair perfectly smooth and even.

To check that a one-length cut is even ask the client to slowly move their head from side to side and backwards and forwards. Any unevenness or long ends will be clearly visible.

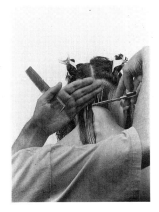
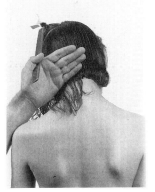
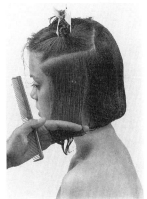

| 1 Back view | 2 Back view | 3 Side view |

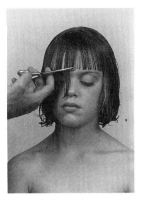
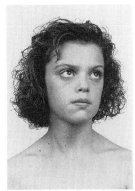

| 4 Front view | 5 Finished result |

The layer cut

In a basic layer cut all sections of the hair are the same length. The outline shape is cut first, and then the inner shape is cut by holding the hair up at 90°.

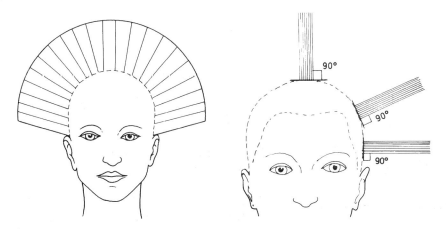

To check that the cut is even, comb the layers in the opposite direction to the way in which you have cut them. They must be perfectly even, with no long ends.

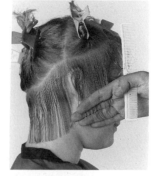

1 Base line: back

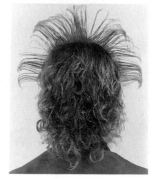

2 Base line: side

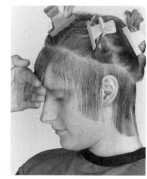

3 Base line: front

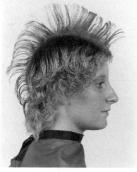

4 Vertical section: 90°

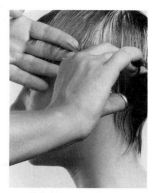

5 Vertical section: 90°

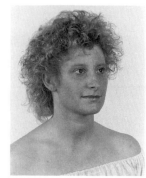

6 Finished result

The graduation

A short graduation cut

In this cut, the **inner layers** of the hair lengths are **longer** than the outline shape (the outline hair length). It is cut using a combination of a one-length cut and scissor or clipper over comb cut.

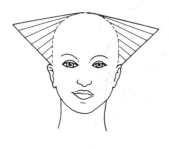

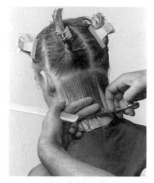

1 Side view

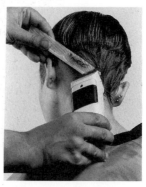

2 Side view

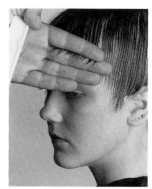

3 Front view

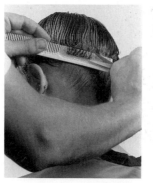

4 Scissors over comb

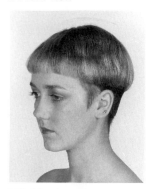

5 Clippers over comb

6 Finished result

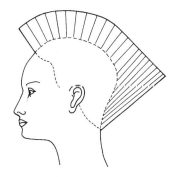

A long graduation cut

This is a long layer cut, in which the **inner layers** of the hair lengths are **shorter** than the outline shape (the outline hair length).

The longer layers have to be **over-directed** (pulled upwards) to match the shorter layers, and then blended together.

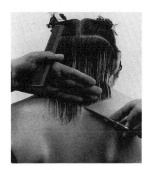

1 Base line: back

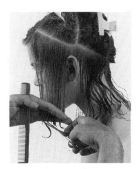

2 Base line: side

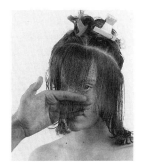

3 Base line: front

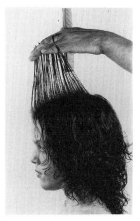

4 Vertical section: front

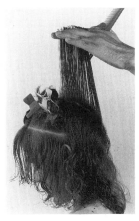

5 Vertical section: back

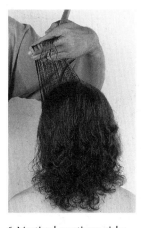

6 Vertical section: side

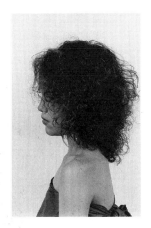

7 Finished result

Variations in cuts

Front lines

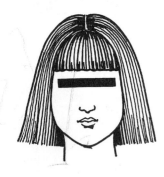 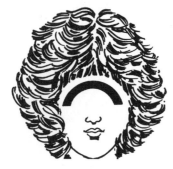 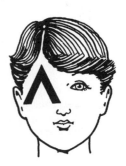 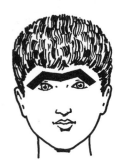

Side lines

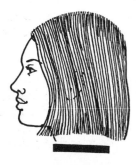 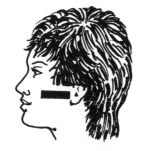 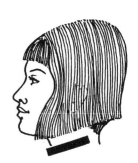

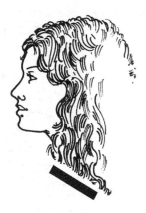 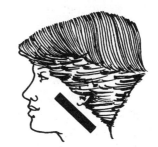 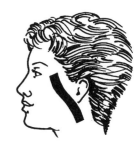

Back lines

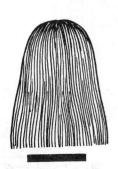 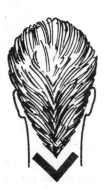 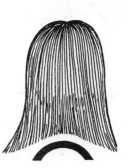 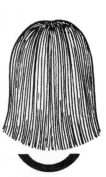 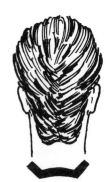

Inside shapes

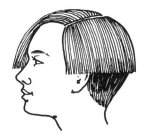 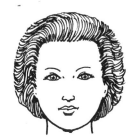 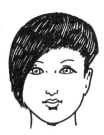 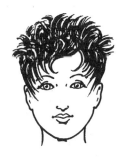

Achieving fashion looks

Once you have mastered the basic cutting methods and techniques you should be able to reproduce any of the latest fashion looks.

A **guideline** or a **baseline** is the cut section of hair that is used as a cutting guide for the next sections. You must always be able to **see the guide** – if you have lost it, it is because the next section was too thick, and you will need to re-section and start again from the guide.

Sometimes there is **more than one guideline**. For instance, with a short graduation, the one-length guideline is cut first – with the fingers resting on the head, the hair is cut to the same length all around the **middle** of the head. For the second guideline the underneath hair is cut at an angle from the nape and the sides, section by section, to meet the first guideline (see short graduation, above).

To **combine** cutting methods, the basic shape of the cut is first produced, often by club cutting, then other methods may be introduced on the same sections of hair to give different looks e.g. a textured, tapered look.

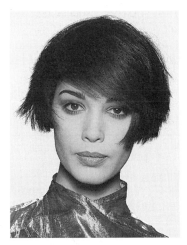 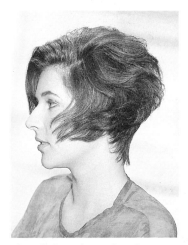

Textured bob   Short bob with two baselines

To do

Find two pictures of different fashion looks for a friend, write up a description of how these were achieved, and why they would be suitable. Describe how a colour or perm would enhance the style.

Accidents when cutting

Accidentally cutting the client

If an accident does happen, **keep calm** and give the client a **sterile dressing**, asking them to apply this with **pressure** to the cut to stop bleeding. (Do not touch the cut yourself because of the health risks, such as AIDS and hepatitis B). Small cuts may be covered with a sterile dressing but larger cuts may need medical attention.

To do

Find out where the first aid box is in your salon and make sure there are plenty of sterile dressings and assorted plasters **before** you start cutting.

Accidentally cutting yourself

Many hairdressers cut themselves during haircutting (a common place is between the first and second fingers, where you hold the hair).

Stop whatever you are doing and excuse yourself from the client. **Rinse the cut** with water to remove any hairs, then **apply pressure** with a **sterile dressing** until the blood clots and the bleeding stops. Dry the area, then apply a sterile plaster.

Test your knowledge

1 When is it better to cut dry hair?
2 What must you remember about the finished hair length when cutting wet hair?
3 Should hair be cut wet or dry when looking for the natural fall?
4 What safety considerations should you take into account when cutting hair?
5 The following are all cutting techniques:
   ■ club cutting
   ■ taper cutting
   ■ pointing and texturising
   ■ scissor/clipper over comb
   ■ thinning.
   Describe the different tools needed for each technique, the type of effect produced and state whether the hair should be cut wet or dry.
6 Why is it important to consult with the client throughout the cutting process?
7 Describe the different cutting angles and how they can be used to achieve a variety of layered looks.

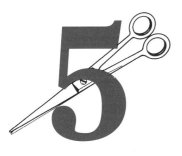

Perming, relaxing and neutralising

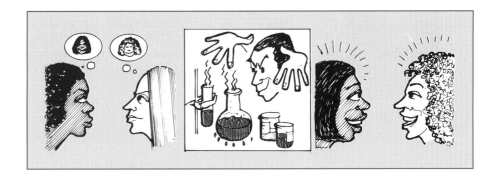

Perming

Permanent waving and curling is a technique used to change the shape of the hair **permanently**. As the hair continues to grow, its natural shape may be seen at the roots or regrowth area.

Gowning up

Gown up the client with a protective gown, cape and towels to protect from perm and neutraliser lotions, both of which can damage clothes and skin.

To do
■ Re-read the section in Chapter 1 on gowning up, then watch someone do this. Make a note of exactly how to gown up for a perm in your salon.

Client consultation for perming

A good perm depends not only on your practical skills but also on your ability to make the **right decisions** about your client's hair, both **before** and **during** perming. Here are some points to help you.

Cutting
Most hair needs some cutting, to remove any perm on the ends, to remove dry brittle ends or simply to re-shape before perming. Some hairdressers prefer to cut before perming, others cut the hair after perming and before styling. It is up to you and your client to decide, but **remember**: hair always appears shorter after perming as the curl lifts the hair up.

Perming tests

Always check the scalp for cuts and abrasions before perming as the chemicals can very severely affect these. Small cuts and abrasions can be **protected** with collodian (New-Skin).

To do

■ Re-read the sections in Chapter 1 on pre-perm test curls, elasticity tests, strand tests, porosity tests and incompatibility tests. These are all relevant to perming and relaxing. Make brief notes about how to do each one.

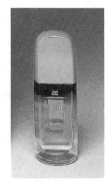

Perming coloured and bleached hair

Hair that has been permanently coloured or bleached is more porous and will absorb perm lotion very quickly. You must, therefore, choose a strength of lotion especially for this type of hair (often No. 2, 3 or 4 strength: refer to the manufacturer's instructions).

Some hair is unevenly porous (e.g. very dry ends) and will need a pre-perm lotion applied to those areas of hair. Pre-perm lotions are applied to towel-dried hair and left on; they are not rinsed out before perming.

Explaining costs

The client will want to know why some perm lotions cost more than others, so you will have to be able to explain the benefits of each. Here are some possible reasons:

- It is a good, strong lotion and will last longer.
- It contains special conditioning agents to keep hair shiny.
- It is a type of acid perm, which breaks down fewer bonds in the hair during processing and so does less damage.

The chemical process of perming

You will need to understand the chemical process so you are able to select the correct type of lotion for your client's hair.

There are three stages in perming:

1. **Softening** – the hair is softened by the perm lotion.
2. **Moulding** – the lotion causes the hair to take up its new shape whilst it is wound around the perm rods.
3. **Fixing** – the hair is fixed permanently into its new shape using neutraliser.

To do

■ Re-read the section in Chapter 1 on hair structure, especially the cuticle and the cortex, and make notes of the differences between the temporary and the permanent bonds.

Softening and moulding the hair during perming

The strong disulphide bonds in the hair are made of an amino acid called **cystine** – these are the bonds that are broken by the perm lotion during the perming process. These bonds are broken because alkaline perm lotions contain a **reducing agent** called **ammonium thioglycollate** (you can smell the ammonia when you open the bottle). As the perm lotion soaks through the cuticle scales and enters the cortex, the reducing agent adds hydrogen to the disulphide bonds, to form a new amino acid, **cysteine**. The hair is now softened and will mould itself to the shape of the perm rods.

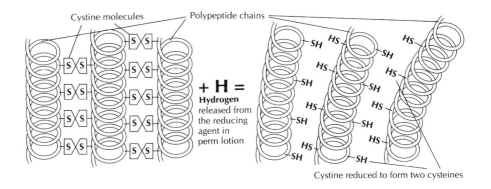

Breaking the disulphide bonds

Hair moulded into shape around the perm rod

To do

■ Re-read the section in Chapter 2 on the pH scale, and make notes on the effect of acids and alkalis on the hair.

Choosing an acid or an alkaline perm

Alkaline perms

These have a pH of approximately 9.5, which opens up the cuticle scales, make the hair more porous, and allows the perm lotion to enter the cortex.

The **higher** the perm lotion's pH, the **more damaging** it is to the hair.

This is why conditioning agents are added to alkaline perms – and why acid perms are becoming increasingly popular. However, alkaline perms are the usual choice for both **normal** and **virgin** hair.

Acid perms

These have activators added to them and rely on heat to open up the cuticle scales so that they can penetrate the cortex. They generally have a slightly acid pH (5.5–7) and contain a chemical called **glyceryl monothioglycollate**.

Fewer bonds in the hair are broken by acid perms, which is why they are said to be better for use on fragile, damaged hair and hair that is easy to process.

Matching hair type to perm lotion

> **To do**
>
> Find out:
>
> - what perm lotions your salon has to offer
> - how many strengths are available
> - the price of each.

Perm lotions are made for many different types of hair:

- **resistant** – non-porous, fine hair which often dries very quickly, or some types of coarse white hair
- **normal** – virgin hair that has not been treated with chemicals
- **tinted** – hair that has been processed with permanent tints
- **bleached** – hair that has been processed with bleach (including highlights)
- **over-porous** – hair that is in a very dry, porous condition.

Hair that is generally **more porous** needs a **weaker** perm lotion and **resistant** hair needs a **stronger** perm lotion.

> **Remember**
>
> Acid perms are particularly good for damaged hair.

> **To do**
>
> - Find out the benefits of each of the different types of perm lotions in your salon.

Perming equipment

Perm rods

Many types of perm rods are available. The most common ones have rubber bands for fastening but Molten permers are also frequently used.

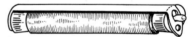

Perm rod fastened

Rods are available in many sizes and are colour-coded so that the sizes can be easily recognised.

> **Remember**
>
> The **larger** the rod the **softer** the curl. The **smaller** the rod the **tighter** the curl.

> **To do**
>
> - Find out all the colours of perm rods available in your salon and compare all the sizes, from the smallest to the largest.

Always wash, rinse and dry perm rods after use. Use a little talcum powder on the rubbers after drying to stop them from perishing.

End papers
These are specially designed, absorbent papers that **make winding easier** and help to **prevent 'fish hooks'** or buckled ends.

Barrier creams
These are thick, heavy, protective creams that should be applied to the client's hairline if they are sensitive to perm lotion. The cream acts as a barrier.

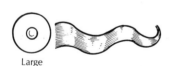

Large

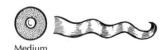

Medium

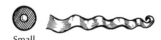

Small

Effect of different rod sizes

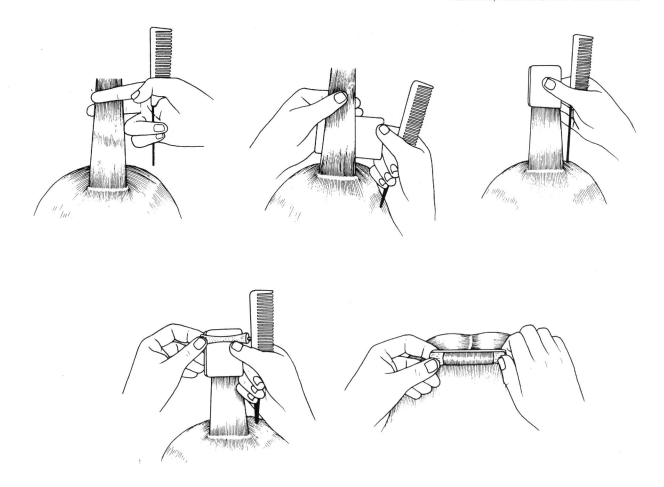

Applying end papers

Always use barrier cream or Vaseline before straightening hair – the chemicals are very strong and can burn both skin and scalp.

Cotton wool

Cotton wool strips must be pre-dampened with warm water to **prevent perm lotion** (and neutraliser) **being absorbed** during use. Place them around the client's hairline to prevent any lotion from running into their eyes, ears or neck. If the cotton wool has absorbed any lotion during processing, replace it immediately to prevent skin burns.

Cotton wool is also used to **absorb excess moisture** from the curlers before the neutraliser is applied.

Protective gloves

These should always be worn when applying perm lotion and neutraliser. If they are difficult to put on because your hands are damp, sprinkle some talcum powder inside them.

Perm caps

Plastic caps are used on the client's hair during processing. They aid development by containing the client's **body heat.**

Accelerators and hood dryers
Many perm lotions need extra heat to make them work. Use either a hood dryer (with a perm cap) or an accelerator in these cases.

To do

Check the manufacturer's instructions on all the perm lotions in your salon to see:

- which perms need heat
- which perms need a plastic cap
- what the recommended development time is.

Perming method

Shampooing
The hair should be shampooed with a plain **soapless shampoo** that contains no extra additives such as conditioner or medicated ingredients. These additives would act as a barrier or film on the hair, and prevent the perm lotion from entering the hair shaft. For the same reason, it is not normal procedure to use a conditioner before perming (unless you are using a specialist pre-perm product).

Towel drying the hair before perming
Once you have combed the hair thoroughly to remove all tangles, then you must towel it dry to prevent the perm lotion from becoming diluted. Use a dry towel and gently squeeze the hair between the two sides of the towel.

The hair should be left wet, but not dripping with water. Since hair is absorbent it must be kept slightly damp so that it does not absorb perm lotion too quickly. In case the hair does dry out too much during winding, keep a water spray nearby to dampen it down.

Sectioning
Sectioning is very important when you are learning to perm – it enables you to work quickly and without being muddled, and to see the size of the rods already used.

There are many different methods of sectioning but the most common is the traditional **nine-section method**.

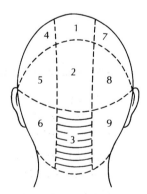

- Start at the front hairline and make sure that section 1 is in the centre, and parallel. It should end just before the crown area.

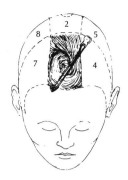

- Always measure the size of the sections against the length of the perm rod – the section should be just a little smaller.
- Secure each section with a section clip or a butterfly clamp, neatly on its own base.
- Continue with section 2, ending level with the top of the ear.
- Now complete section 3 down to the nape.
- Check that sections 1, 2 and 3 are in the centre of the head, not lop-sided.
- Continue with section 4, measuring both the top and bottom of the section with the perm rod.
- To complete sections 5 and 6, section from the top of section 3 across to the top of the ear, level with the bottom of section 4.

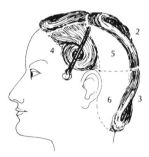

- Repeat sections 4, 5 and 6 on the opposite side of the head to complete sections 7, 8 and 9.

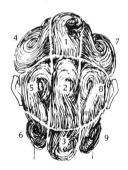

To do
■ Practise sectioning on models who have time to spare, but are actually having a shampoo and set or blow dry.

Sub-sectioning
Sub-sections are the **smaller sections** taken for each individual perm rod.

The length of the perm rod decides the size of the large section, but the **depth or width** of the rod dictates the **size of the sub-section**.

Each sub-section must be parallel, or uneven winding will result.

Remember

Always ask the client to position their head correctly (forwards, upright or sideways) for you so that you can work properly.

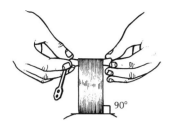

Winding hair at 90°

Once the hair has been sub-sectioned, the hair should be combed smoothly at an angle of 90° away from the head.

Winding the curlers

Use a pin-tail comb to wind the ends around the rod, using end papers if necessary to prevent 'fish hooks'.

Always keep the perm rod parallel to the head during winding or it will not sit properly on its base (the sub-section).

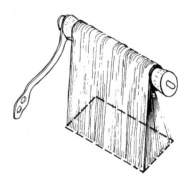

Remember

Always wind the hair evenly, without causing **undue tension** or pulling on the hair.

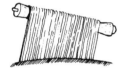

Non-parallel winding

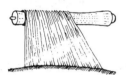

Lop-sided winding

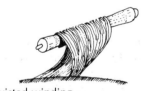

Twisted winding

As clients' heads are round (not square) and the perm rods are straight, perfect winding is difficult to achieve without practice.

To do

Practise perm winding using water on model heads (or models).

- Check that the size of the rods is correct for the length of hair and curl required.
- Check the number of rods to be used (the normal amount is 60–80 per head).
- Time yourself: try to complete the wind in 30–40 minutes.

Remember

When fastening the rubbers to the perm rods make sure they are not twisted. If they cut into the hair when the perm is processing the hair will break off.

Result of perming with rubbers fixed too tightly

Winding variations

Directional winding
This is where the hair is wound in the direction of the **finished style**.

Directional winding

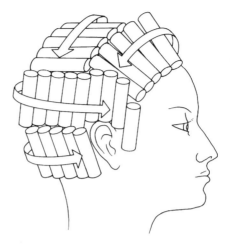

Brick winding
This technique gives a more **uniform curl** and **avoids partings** in the finished result.

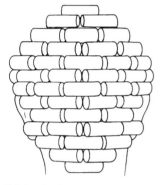

Brick winding

Applying perm lotion

Pre-damping
This is when the hair is lotioned **after sectioning** and during sub-sectioning. This technique is often used for resistant (non-porous) or for long hair.

Post-damping
This is when the lotion is applied **after winding** has been completed, and applicator bottles with special nozzles are often used.

Safety points to remember
- Wear your **gloves** when applying lotion to the hair.
- Applying lotion can be very **dangerous**, as it can easily run into the client's eyes. If this does happen, **rinse immediately** with cold water on a pad of cotton wool until the client says the stinging has stopped.
- Always use a strip of **dampened cotton wool** around the hairline and hold a piece of cotton wool during lotioning to use for absorbing any excess.
- **Pull burns** may result if the hair is wound tightly – the neck of the hair follicle opens, allowing perm lotion to enter. If the scalp is scratched this irritation could become infected, causing **folliculitis**.

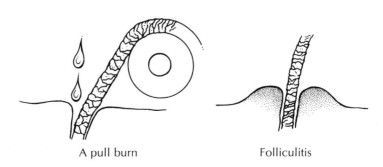

A pull burn   Folliculitis

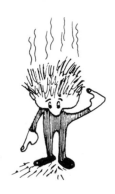

- Many manufacturers' bottles of perm lotion and neutraliser look very similar. To avoid applying the **wrong lotion** do not get the bottle of neutraliser out until you are ready to neutralise.

Processing and timing the perm

The timing of the moulding stage, where the hair is softened around the perm rods, is crucial. If the lotion is left on too long then the hair will become over-processed, frizzy and break off.

To do
■ Re-read the section in Chapter 1 on a development test curl and practise as often as possible.

The length of time the perm lotion is left on will vary according to:

- The **room temperature** – heat speeds up chemical reactions, so the hotter the room is the quicker it will work.
- The **porosity** of the hair – the more porous the hair the quicker the reaction.
- The client's **body heat** – if the head is covered with a perm cap, the body heat will be trapped in and the perm will process more quickly.
- The **strength** of the perm lotion – the stronger the perm lotion the quicker it will act.
- The **pH** of the perm lotion – generally the higher the pH, the quicker the reaction.
- Remember – the neutralising processes will stop any further development of the perm lotion.

Remember
Never leave your client during processing. Keep checking every few minutes, especially with porous, bleached hair.

Two-stage curly perms

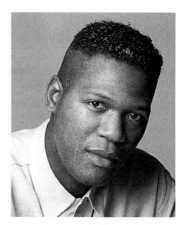

Afro perms, sometimes called 'wet look' or 'curly' perms, are possible on afro hair because they chemically **straighten** or **relax the curly hair first** using a **curl rearranger**. The hair is then permed with a weaker perm lotion, a **curl booster**, into larger, softer curls.

Curl rearrangers may be available in **three or four different strengths**, but **curl boosters** are available in only **one strength**.

Method

- The **curl rearranger** is **applied** to the hair after a light pre-perm shampoo.
- The hair is towel dried, given a **pre-conditioning treatment** (a protective

polymer), covered with a plastic cap and processed under a cool dryer for ten minutes.

- Always **protect the client's skin around the hairline** with barrier cream or Vaseline.
- The product is **applied in the same way as a tint or a bleach**, section by section.
- The hair is then **combed straight**, gently but firmly.
- The re-arranger is then **developed** according to the manufacturer's directions, taking 10–30 minutes, **until the hair becomes less curly** and is smooth, straight, and pliable.
- The hair is thoroughly **rinsed** then **blotted dry** with a towel, taking care **not to tangle** the hair.
- **Curly perms are then wound on perm rods** and a **curl booster is applied** either before winding (pre-damped) or after winding (post-damped).
- The hair is then **processed** in the normal manner.
- After perming, the hair is **neutralised** according to the manufacturer's instructions.

The curl rearrangers and boosters are **thioglycollate** chemicals. They swell the hair shaft and break down some of the disulphide bonds.

If a **wet look** is desired use a **glycerine-based activator/moisturiser**.

> **Remember**
>
> **Never** perm afro hair that is badly damaged or has been **chemically relaxed** previously. If in doubt, take a pre-perm test curl.

Relaxing or permanently straightening hair

Relaxers are very popular with clients who have excessively curly or wavy hair because once their hair is **permanently straightened** they have a much **wider choice** of hairstyles. It also takes the pain out of combing their hair.

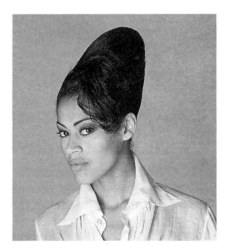

> **To do**
>
> ■ Re-read the section in Chapter 1 on Afro hair structure.

Tight curly **afro hair** has **more cuticle scales** and is **initially more difficult** to chemically process.

Relaxing creams are **extremely alkaline**, with a pH of 10–14, which means they are very strong chemicals.

To remove curl

Sodium hydroxide relaxers (caustic soda, sometimes called lye) are the strongest and fastest-acting chemicals.

Calcium hydroxide (occasionally **potassium hydroxide** or **guanidine hydroxide**) relaxers (sometimes called no-lye) are **not as strong** and **do not require the scalp to be based** before application. These relaxers are often available for home use as they are **not as effective as other relaxers.** However, they do tend to lighten the colour, causing a reddish tinge, and leave the hair more dry and brittle.

Both of these straightening chemicals permanently change the structure of the hair by changing one-third of the **cystine** bonds into new **lanthionine** bonds (with one sulphur atom), which keep the hair straight. This process is **stopped** (sometimes known as **hydrolysis**) by a **neutralising shampoo**. The low pH of this shampoo stops any further chemical action.

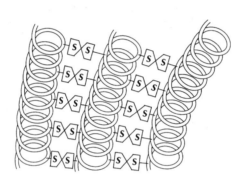

New single sulphur lanthionine bonds formed, keeping the hair straight

Tight curly/wavy hair with disulphide bonds intact

After being shaped with straightening cream, processed and having neutralising shampoo applied

To reduce the degree of curl

Ammonium thioglycollate, the same chemical that is used to perm hair and make it curly, may also be used to straighten fine difficult hair, or if the client doesn't want all the curl removed.

These **'thio' straighteners** may be either a **thick cream**, which is used in exactly the same way as the hydroxide relaxers (i.e. the hair is smoothed straight), or **normal perm lotion** that is combed onto the hair and then **wound around large rollers**.

Ammonium thioglycollate breaks down the disulphide bonds (by using a reducing agent – hydrogen), and changes the cystine in the hair to cysteine.

Both the cream and liquid processes are **stopped** by an **oxidising neutraliser** which reforms the broken disulphide bonds and holds the hair in its new shape.

> **Remember**
>
> Sodium and calcium **hydroxide relaxers** and **ammonium thioglycollate straighteners** and perms are **incompatible** – they do not work with each other. All the hair must grow out and be cut off before changing from one to the other.

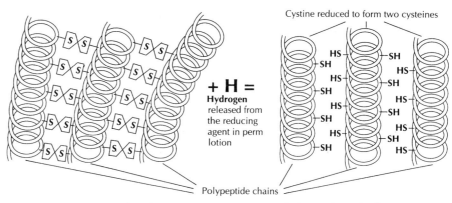

Cystine reduced to form two cysteines

+ H =
Hydrogen
released from
the reducing
agent in perm
lotion

Polypeptide chains

Breaking the disulphide bonds

Hair moulded into shape by being combed straight with straightening cream

Matching relaxer to hair type

- **Fine**, **tinted or lightened** hair (hair that has been previously chemically treated) – use mild relaxers.
- **Normal, medium-textured virgin hair** – use regular relaxers.
- **Coarse, virgin hair** – use strong or super-relaxers.

Precautions

To do

Re-read the sections in Chapter 1 on strand tests, elasticity tests, porosity tests and incompatibility tests.

Check

- The **client's scalp** for any soreness, cuts, abrasions or disorders. If in doubt do not proceed – call your supervisor. Leave 72 hours between tinting/bleaching and relaxing treatments.
- The **client's hair condition** for:
  - **elasticity and tensile strength** (elasticity test)
  - **tightness of curl** (strand test i.e. product strength and timing).
  - **texture and porosity** (porosity test)
  - **previous chemical processes** (incompatibility test)
  - any **breakage** (elasticity test).

  If you are in any doubt, proceed with the necessary test, and suggest some reconditioning treatments.
- The **client's record card** for any previous treatments.
- Exactly what **degree of straightness** the client requires (use photographs from the style books).

To do

■ Take three cuttings each of tight curly and wavy hair and strand test them with a sodium hydroxide, calcium hydroxide and ammonium thioglycollate relaxer. Make a note of the development times and any differences in the elasticity and condition of the hair.

Points to remember

Relaxers are very strong chemicals.

- Make sure that you have **sufficient product knowledge**. Try writing out the manufacturer's instructions in your own words and checking with your supervisor.

Remember

If in doubt choose a weaker product and then apply a stronger product if the process is rather slow.

Remember

The scalp is very sensitive after either cane row or extensions have been removed. **Do not** chemically relax hair on the same day that they are removed.

- If the product **touches the scalp or skin for a prolonged period** it will cause serious **irritation, burning** and **damage**. If the client complains that her skin or scalp are 'burning' **rinse the relaxer off immediately** and use the neutralising shampoo.
- Always use the **back wash-basin** to remove the relaxer and for applying the neutralising shampoo.
- If the **relaxer accidentally enters the eye** it could cause **blindness**, so shield the unaffected eye with one hand, and **flush the affected eye** with lots of water. Seek medical help if the irritation persists.
- If the product **stays in contact with the hair for too long** the hair may become **brittle, break off** or even **dissolve**. **Do not relax the hair if you think there will be any hair breakage**.
- **Never apply the product to hair that has already been relaxed** – apply it only to new regrowth.
- Make sure that you are using the **correct straightening chemical** for the hair, and the **correct strength** of chemical. If in doubt, check with your supervisor.
- **Never** use any **additional heat** (from hairdryers or accelerators or steamers) when processing sodium or calcium **hydroxide** relaxers – they develop very quickly and could dissolve the hair.
- **Always** wear rubber gloves, and gown up your client properly.
- Always **protect** the client's hairline and scalp by applying Vaseline or special basing cream.
- **Never mix** relaxers, neutralisers and other products from **different manufacturers** – they are unlikely to work together. **If the hair becomes damaged you will be legally responsible.**
- Keep record cards up to date.

Method

1. **Gown up** as for perming.
2. **Do not shampoo** the hair or brush the scalp. Apply the **basing cream** or Vaseline to the scalp area section by section (like a tint). **Place the cream**, do not press or rub it in, as it **must not cover the hair**.
3. **Check the manufacturer's instructions, and wear gloves.** If a special conditioner (filler) needs to be used, apply it evenly at this stage and blot off any excess
4. **Section** the hair **into four** and then prepare **sub-sections**.

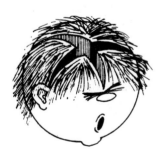

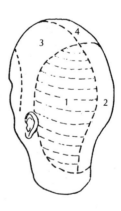

5. Start at the nape area, taking small sections and applying relaxer cream either with the back of the comb or a brush, avoiding the scalp area. Apply to the front hairline, where the hair is more porous, last.

6. **Smooth the hair straight** with your gloved hand to spread the product. **Cross-check** the application in the opposite direction, reapplying relaxer to any uncovered areas.
7. **With previously straightened hair apply to the regrowth only, taking care not to overlap onto the previously straightened hair.**
8. **Leave the hair as straight as possible. Do not continually comb the hair** – it may easily break.
9. **Develop the product according to the manufacturer's instructions.** This may take 2–18 minutes. Check it continually. It is ready when you remove some of the product from a strand and let the hair relax with your comb to see the degree of straightness.
10. When processing is complete **rinse at a back wash-basin with a strong stream of warm water**. Start at the hairline and let the force of the water remove the cream. Do not use your hands. Rinse until the water runs clear. Some manufacturers advise the use of a reconstructor at this stage, which should be left for five minutes before the **neutralising shampoo** is applied.

Perming and relaxing faults and corrections

Fault	Causes	Correction
The perm is not curly enough	Poor shampooing (hair greasy) Poor neutralising Perm rods too large Too few perm rods used Perm lotion too weak Not enough perm lotion applied Perm lotion not left on long enough	Re-perm the hair using a weaker perm lotion
Straight pieces of hair	Sections too wide Incorrect angling and placing of perm rods Carelessly leaving out pieces of hair	Re-perm straight pieces of hair, but clip the rest of the hair well away from the perm lotion
Hair too curly	Perm rods used were too small	May be gently relaxed by a senior stylist
Over-processed hair (looks frizzy when wet and straight when dry)	Perm lotion too strong Too much heat used during processing Too much tension used Rods too small	Suggest a course of conditioning treatments and regular haircuts. Do not re-perm the hair: it will break off
'Fish hooks' or buckled ends	Poor winding; ends not smoothly wound around the perm rod	These must be cut off
Scalp/skin damage or irritation	Perm lotion or relaxers coming into contact with scalp/skin – if it enters the hair follicle 'pull burns' occur Barrier cream not applied to sensitive skin areas Cuts and abrasions to the scalp	Remove any excess perm lotion or relaxers with water. Apply a soothing moisturising cream to the area
Hair breakage	Too much tension during winding Rubber too tight or twisted Perm lotion or relaxing product too strong Hair over processed	Suggest a course of reconditioning treatments or restructurants

Neutralising

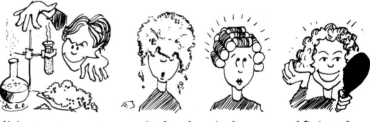

Neutralising permanent waves is the chemical process of **fixing the new curl** in the hair. It is a very important process. If it is not done properly then the curl will 'drop', the perm will relax, and the hair will become straighter.

Once the 'S'-shaped movement has been formed in the hair, the processing is complete and the hair should be neutralised.

'S'-shape to curler size

To do

■ Watch an experienced person in your salon neutralising a perm and make notes on the procedure.

The chemical process of neutralising

The neutralising process is sometimes called **normalising** (returning the hair back to normal), and sometimes called **oxidising** (because oxygen is added during the process).

The chemical process of neutralising is an **oxidation process** – all neutralisers contain **oxygen**. The active ingredient in the neutraliser which gives off the oxygen is a weak solution of **hydrogen peroxide** or **sodium bromate**.

The oxygen combines with the hydrogen (which has been released from the reducing agent in perm lotion) to form water. This is why the hair takes longer to dry after a perm: it contains so much water.

The **disulphide bonds** rejoin in their new permed shape. At the same time the two cysteine molecules become cystine molecules again.

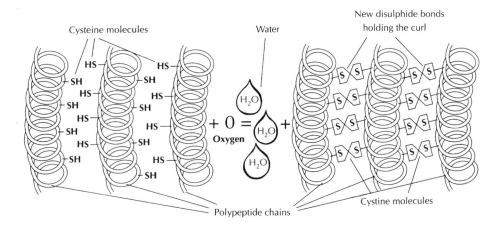

Disulphide bonds broken
by perm lotion

Hair fixed in its new curled
shape

To do

■ Read the manufacturer's instructions on some neutraliser in your salon and make notes on the ingredients.

Rinsing the hair before applying neutraliser

Take the client to the wash-basin (a back wash-basin is preferable as there is less likelihood of chemicals running into the client's eyes), and make sure the client is both comfortable and correctly gowned for neutralising (sometimes a protective disposable plastic cape is used around the shoulders).

Test the water temperature on the inside of your wrist and check the temperature during rinsing by keeping one of your fingers under the water spray. Ask the client if the temperature is comfortable, then make sure you thoroughly rinse all the curlers on the head. Use your free hand to cup the water over the rods and let it run back down into the wash-basin. Continue rinsing until all the perm solution has been rinsed out of the hair. This will take a minimum of 5 minutes.

Removing excess water from the wound hair

This is also called 'blotting' the hair and should always be done **before** the neutraliser is applied. Use either a dry absorbent towel or a wad of cotton wool and press carefully into the rods so as not to disturb them. Remember the hair is still very soft and fragile at this stage.

Up to 60 ml of water can be removed during 'blotting', so do it thoroughly.

Mixing the neutraliser

To do

- Check the manufacturer's instructions on all of the neutralisers in your salon. Make notes on the mixing and timing.

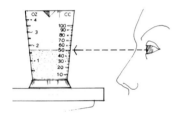

- Always make sure you have the **correct neutraliser** for the perm that has been used (and that you have not picked up the perm lotion by mistake).
- Some neutralisers have to be measured out or need mixing, so always check the **amounts** needed.
- Make sure you have the **correct equipment** with which to apply the neutraliser. Some lotions are foamed up in a large bowl with a neutraliser sponge, some are applied to the hair then foamed up with a sponge on the rods, others are poured directly on to the hair from a bottle with a special applicator nozzle.

Applying the neutraliser

The neutraliser must be thoroughly applied so that every single rod is covered with the solution. You will normally need to use about two-thirds of the amount, saving the last third to use once the rods have been removed from the hair.

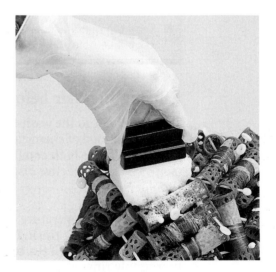

Timing

Most neutralisers are left on for about five minutes. The timing is very important. If you are not sure either check the manufacturer's instructions again or ask your supervisor. **If the neutraliser is not left on long enough, the disulphide bonds will not have time to reform and the hair will go straight.**

Unwinding the curlers

When the oxidation is complete (after 5 minutes) each rod should be **gently removed** without applying any tension or pulling the hair. Always start removing the rods from underneath, at the nape area and work carefully, removing one rod at a time.

You can now apply the **remaining neutraliser** (one-third of the original amount) to the ends of the hair. To make sure that all the hair has absorbed the neutraliser solution, **leave it on** for a few more minutes while you rinse and dry the perm rods and dispose of the end papers.

Rinsing the hair after neutralising

Test the temperature of the water – remember that the client's scalp may be a little tender; so do not have the water too hot.

Rinse the hair thoroughly and apply an anti-oxy conditioner to prevent **creeping oxidation**.

An acid-balanced conditioner is helpful after perming to return the hair to its normal pH-balanced, acid state.

Effect on colour

Sometimes neutralisers have the effect of **lightening** or **fading hair colour**. This happens particularly if the hair is porous or has been permanently coloured (tinted). The easiest remedy is to use a matching temporary or semi-permanent colour, but check with your supervisor which colour would be best.

Neutralising shampoos for relaxers

Shampoo the hair thoroughly to remove excess relaxers from the hair and scalp and to stop the action of the relaxer.

On the **second shampoo, firmly comb the hair straight** – but be gentle on the scalp.

Leave for **five minutes**, then rinse thoroughly.

Check the manufacturer's instructions – some products change colour to show that the neutralising is complete.

Blot the hair, then use a **pH-balanced moisturising conditioner** as a treatment and **leave for ten minutes**, then **rinse thoroughly**.

Remember

The hair is still in a softened state so **never pull** the rods out of the hair. Always work gently or you will straighten the perm.

Remember

Neutralising shampoos work differently from perm neutralisers.
Never use a neutralising shampoo after a normal perm, or a perm neutraliser after straightening hair.

1 Give two other names for the chemical process of neutralising.
2 What does the oxygen from the neutraliser form in the hair during the 'fixing stage'.
3 What happens to the cysteine molecules during neutralising?
4 Why is it important to time both the rinsing (the removal of perm lotion) and the neutraliser product?
5 Why is it important to unwind the perm rods gently?
6 Name the two chemical ingredients often found in neutralisers.
7 What can happen to the hair colour during neutralising?
8 List the causes of scalp or skin damage or irritation and how they can be corrected.
9 What is the effect of using a neutralising shampoo on hair that has just been relaxed?
10 Why is it important that neutralising shampoos, not perming neutralisers, are used after relaxing?
11 Why is it important to time the neutralising shampoo?
12 Why must the hair be combed straight on the second neutralising shampoo?

Record cards

Remember

Always check the name **and** address of the client: you may have ten clients called 'Mrs Brown'.

The perming record card is normally completed after perming but before styling and should then be filed away.

Permanent waving record card

Client name:

Address:

Daytime tel. no.:

Date of 1st perm: _____

Colour treated or natural: _____

If treated, product: _____

Texture: _____

Condition: _____

Date	Type of lotion	Lotion strength	Size of curlers	Result required	Development time and method	Special notes	Neutralising time and method	Conditioner	Result obtained	Stylist

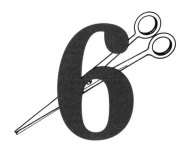

Colouring and bleaching

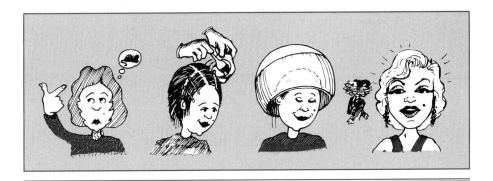

Colouring and bleaching hair are a very exciting part of hairdressing. You can change the client's hair colour quite subtly just by covering a few grey hairs, or very dramatically by turning a mousy brown into a glamorous blonde!

Many hairdressers are frightened of applying colour because they do not understand the theory behind it. For instance:

- You cannot put a light ash blonde tint on a dark brown head of hair and expect it to come out blonde. You need to bleach it first.
- You cannot put a rich auburn colour on a client with a head of naturally white hair; their hair will turn out a **very** bright red. You need to mix in some brown with the rich auburn colour.

To do

Find the colour charts in your salon and ask your supervisor which ones are:

- temporary colours
- semi-permanent colours
- permanent colours.

Make a note of each for future use.

Establishing hair colour

Lighting

Light plays a very important part in the appearance of hair colours. If you are sitting in a darkened room such as a cinema, then you cannot see the true colour of the hair of the person next to you until the lights come on.

In the same way you cannot see the true colour of your client's hair if you do not have good lighting in your salon.

The best light in which to look at hair colour is **natural daylight**. If your salon has lots of large windows and white walls, then you should be able to see hair colour quite well.

However, if the salon has lots of dark walls or poor lighting, then you may have to take the client over to a window or show them the true colour (especially coppers and reds) with a hand mirror.

HEALTH MATTERS

Assessing the client's hair colour is a critical part of hair colouring, so try to organise your workstation without glare so that you are not looking directly into the light, at a white wall or a mirror reflecting either. Glare can be both irritating and tiring to your eyes.

Natural hair colour

There are two types of natural hair colour.

White hair

This contains no colour pigments at all. Remember there is no such thing as grey hair – it is white hair mixed with naturally coloured hair. For example, light brown hair and white hair looks salt and pepper colour, dark brown hair and white hair looks steel grey.

Naturally coloured hair

This contains colour pigments found in the cortex. It is known as 'virgin hair', which means that it has never been artificially coloured.

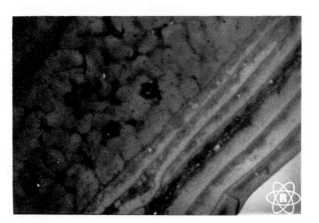

Colour pigments in the cortex

Hair pigment

The two main types of pigment found in hair are:

- **melanin** (sometimes called **granular pigment**), which is brown or black
- **pheomelanin** (sometimes called **diffuse pigment**), which is red or yellow.

All natural hair colours are made up of a combination of these colours. For example:

- **medium brown** hair has lots of brown and a little black, red and yellow
- **coppery red** hair has lots of red and yellow and a little brown and black
- **blonde** hair has lots of yellow and a very little red and brown.

To **change the colour** of hair, new pigments are added: sometimes to the surface of the hair (temporary and semi-permanent colours), and sometimes to the hair cortex (permanent colours).

To **lighten** the natural hair colour the pigments are bleached out.

Hair texture and porosity related to hair colour

Hair that is more **porous** because it has been permed, relaxed or highlighted, or that is in a generally damaged condition, will **absorb colour more quickly** in some areas – giving an **uneven** colour as a result. Remember also that colours will **fade** more quickly on porous hair.

Very **coarse** textured hair (such as strong white hair) can be **resistant to colour** so you may need to do a test cutting.

To do

- Re-read the section in Chapter 1 on porosity tests and test cuttings.

Choosing the right colour

Skin tones

Younger clients generally have fuller, plumper skin without lines and wrinkles. The skin of older clients has undergone changes in shape and texture and may also have lost colour. Very few older people have naturally rosy cheeks; any redness is often due to broken veins or cosmetic make-up. Young people can therefore colour their hair most colours and look good (the only exception is the range of red colours, which should not be used on clients with red skin tones).

Dark or ashen colours can be very ageing on older clients. They may wish to return their hair to its natural colour in order to look younger, but this is not usually successful as the colour they had then may not always suit them now.

Shade and depth of colour

You will have to learn to train your eye to look at hair colours for two things:

- The **depth of colour**. This is how light or how dark the hair is – very light blonde, blonde, light brown, medium brown, etc. This is also called the **base shade**.
- The **tone of colour**. This is the shade of colour on a particular depth – light ash blonde, light golden blonde, light warm blonde, light silver blonde.

The International Colour Chart System (ICC)

Most manufacturers use a numbering system called the 'International Colour Chart System' for choosing colours. This is so that hairdressers can be precise when choosing colours. For example, your idea of red may be a rich auburn colour, but your client's idea of red may be a pale copper colour, so you will need to use a colour chart to achieve exactly the colour your client wants.

Below is an example of an ICC chart. You can see that the **depth** of colours (or base colours) are numbered from **1 to 10** and the **tones** of colours are numbered as **.1, .2, .3, .4, .5, .6**. Some examples are already written in, e.g. 9.1 is a very light ash blonde, because 9 is a very light blonde and .1 is ash.

Example of an ICC chart

Tone (shades of the basic colour) →

Depth (base colours)

Tone / Depth	.1 (Blue) Ash	.2 (Violet) Mauve Ash	.3 (Yellow) Gold	.4 (Orange) Warm	.5/.6 (Red) Red	(Green) Matt Concentrate Colour
10 Lightest blonde						
9 Very light blonde	e.g. very light ash blonde 9.1					
8 Light blonde						
7 Blonde			e.g. golden blonde 7.3			
6 Dark blonde						
5 Light brown				e.g. light warm brown 5.4		
4 Brown						
3 Dark brown						
2 Very dark brown						
1 Black						

Extra information
Some colours have two numbers after the depth, e.g. 8.31, 9.33, 6.01.

- The **first number after the point** is the **strongest tone**, e.g. 8.31 is light golden blonde (the 8 and the 3) with a little ash tone (the 1).
- If the **second number after the point** is the **same** number as the first, then the tone is **twice as concentrated** (twice as bright) – e.g. 9.33.
- If the **first number after the point** is a 0, e.g. 6.01, then the tone is **diluted**, e.g. dark natural ash blonde.

Not all manufacturers list their colour tones as numbers: some have letters such as G for Gold, R for Red.

To do

- Try to learn all the names of the colour depths and their numbers on your salon's colour chart.
- Make yourself familiar with all of the colour tones on your salon's colour chart.

Summary of points to remember when choosing a hair colour

Client's requirements
- How light or dark (depth) do they want the colour?
- What tone do they want, e.g. red, copper, ashen?
- Use the shade chart to decide together.

Client's natural (base) colour
Very dark hair cannot be tinted to light blonde (you will have to pre-lighten with bleach).

Amount of white hair present
The more white hair the brighter any warm tones such as red and copper will show up.

Hair condition and porosity
Unevenly porous hair will absorb colours unevenly.

Hair texture and density
Some coarse textured hair is resistant to colouring (take a test cutting first).

Complexion and skin tones
Never colour an older client's hair too dark or too ash – it will make them look older.

The colour spectrum

Light from the sun is made up of a mixture of colours, which can be seen naturally in a rainbow. These colours – red, orange, yellow, green, blue, indigo and violet – make up the colour spectrum.

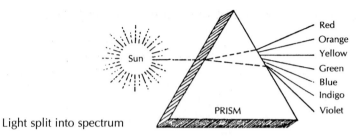

Light split into spectrum

You can see all these colours easily when you look through a cut-glass prism. There is a mnemonic to remember the colours: '**R**ichard **O**f **Y**ork **G**ained **B**attles **I**n **V**ain'.

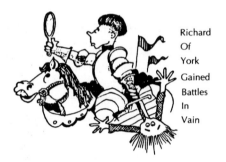

Richard
Of
York
Gained
Battles
In
Vain

These same colours are used as colour pigments in hair colouring. Here is how they are related to the colour **tones** that hairdressers use.

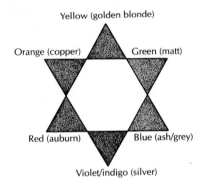

The colour star

For example, you would **not** say to a client 'I'm going to put orange on your hair'; you would say 'I'm going to put a copper tone on your hair'.

You have to know about these tones because the colours **opposite** each other on the star **cancel each other out**. If a client's hair becomes too red you apply green (matt), if a client's hair becomes too orange you apply blue (ash), if it becomes too yellow (this may happen after highlights), you apply violet (silver).

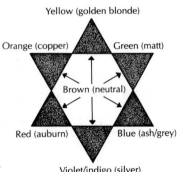

The colour cancellation star

Remember

Yellow discoloration is masked by **purple** (mauve or silver). **Orange** discoloration is masked by **blue** (ash). **Red** discoloration is masked by **green** (matt).

To do

■ Watch some children washing out their paintbrushes after a painting class. All the bright reds, blues, yellows, greens, oranges and mauves will mix together (colour cancellation) to form a sludgy brown or **neutral** colour.

Using hydrogen peroxide for colouring and bleaching

Hydrogen peroxide is mixed with both permanent colours and hair bleaches. If it were used by itself it would **lighten** hair colour and make the hair more **porous**. It is occasionally used to soften very coarse textured hair before applying a permanent tint.

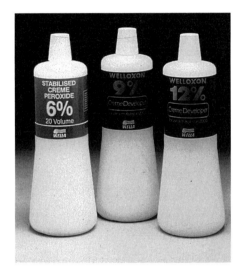

To do

Read the section in Chapter 10 relating to the COSHH Act, and list all the precautions needed when using hydrogen peroxide, bleaches and colour in the salon.

Once it is mixed with permanent colours or hair bleaches, hydrogen peroxide releases oxygen – it is therefore known as an **oxidising agent**. The chemical formula for hydrogen peroxide is H_2O_2, and here you can see how it breaks down during mixing:

H_2O_2 $\xrightarrow{\text{breaks down to form}}$ $H_2O + O$
Hydrogen peroxide   Water and oxygen

Volume strength

Hydrogen peroxide is available in either volume strengths or percentage (%) strengths.

Hydrogen peroxide: strengths and uses

Volume strength (vol.)	Percentage strength (%)	Use
10 vol.	3%	For adding weak colour (e.g. bleach toners)
20 vol.	6%	For adding colour (e.g. for most tinting purposes
30 vol.	9%	For lightening hair colour
40 vol.	12%	For highlights and highlifting tints
60 vol.	18%	For highlights and highlifting tints

It may be supplied as either a liquid or a cream, but the strengths are the same. Hydrogen peroxide will not work if it has 'gone off' which means it has lost its strength (and its oxygen). This will happen if it is not stored properly. Therefore you must always:

- keep the **containers tightly closed** and put the lids back on as soon as possible after use
- **measure out** the amount of peroxide you need. If you have any left over, do **not pour it back into the bottle** as it may have picked up some dust
- store it in a **cool, dark place**.

All peroxides have an acid stabiliser added to them which helps to prevent loss of strength.

Sometimes you might have to dilute liquid hydrogen peroxide from a stronger solution to a weaker one. The table below shows the different dilutions.

Dilution of hydrogen peroxide

Volume of hydrogen peroxide	Parts of hydrogen peroxide		Parts of distilled water	Volume produced
60	2	+	1	40
60	1	+	1	30
60	1	+	2	20
60	1	+	5	10
40	3	+	1	30
40	1	+	1	20
40	1	+	3	10
30	2	+	1	20
30	1	+	2	10
20	1	+	1	10

Preparing the client for colouring or bleaching

> **Remember**
>
> Protect your own clothes with a dye apron and wear rubber gloves.

Gowning up

It is best to gown up the client with a plastic or rubberised bleaching or tinting gown to prevent any chemical splashes reaching the client's clothes. Most salons also use towels, shoulder capes and tissues around the neck area.

When you are using very dark colours or have clients with sensitive skin you may also need to use protective **barrier cream** around the hairline.

To do

■ Re-read the section in Chapter 1 on gowning up and make notes about the various methods.

For **partial head block colouring** section off the hair that is not being coloured and secure it firmly with section clips. Cover the hair that is not to be coloured with strips of cotton wool, either clipped to the hair or attached to a thin film of barrier cream near the roots.

Checking the scalp

Always check the client's scalp for any inflammation, cuts or abrasions. If you are in doubt whether to proceed, call your supervisor and **tactfully** (remember the client's feelings) ask for advice.

Skin test

Make sure your client has had a skin test if 'para' dyes are to be used (see Chapter 1).

Hair texture and porosity

Check the hair texture and porosity. Remember that some coarse-textured hair can be resistant to colour and unevenly porous hair (dry ends) can absorb colour unevenly. Take a test cutting if you are unsure about the result.

Remember

When measuring liquids: 1 fluid ounce = approx. 30 ml.

Record cards

There is quite a lot of information needed when colouring and bleaching a client's hair, so always complete the record card straight away in case you forget any of the details.

Hair colour record card

Client name: _____ Natural hair colour: _____

Address: _____ Texture: _____

_____ Condition: _____

Daytime tel. no.: _____

Skin test: Date: Name of operator:

RECORD OF APPLICATION

Date	Type	Colour	Hydrogen peroxide	Development		Application special notes	Comb through	After treatment	Result		Stylist
				Method	Time				Required	Obtained	

111

Bleaching hair

Hairdressers use bleach to lighten hair when other products such as highlifting tints are not strong enough.

Clients who have naturally 'mousy' hair that lightens in the sunlight may wish to achieve this effect by bleaching. Blonde hair is often considered to be more flattering, especially with sun-tanned skin, and once clients have experienced being blonde they often feel that their own colour is less exciting.

Blonde highlights, especially on layered hair (where the natural coloured regrowth is less obvious), are easier to sell to clients. The initial cost of highlights, especially woven highlights (which take more time) may be high, but they need to be repeated only every few months. If clients prefer a full head bleach then the regrowth must be done every few weeks.

Bleaching materials

Emulsion bleach
Emulsion bleaches are made up of three separate parts:

- an oil or gel bleach
- hydrogen peroxide (normally 20 vol. [6%] or 30 vol. [9%])
- boosters or activators (sachets of powder).

Always check the manufacturer's instructions for the recommended strength of peroxide and the number of boosters or activators to use.

Make sure you mix up in the **correct order**. The peroxide and boosters are generally mixed first and then the oil or gel bleach is added so that it does not become lumpy.

Emulsion bleaches are particularly good for **whole-head** and **regrowth** bleaches as the consistency is easy to apply.

To do

- Look at the emulsion bleach left in the bowl after it has been used and see how much it has expanded due to the release of oxygen.

Powder bleach
Powder bleaches are made of two parts:

- bleach powder
- hydrogen peroxide (normally 20 vol. [6%] or 30 vol. [9%]).

Powder bleaches have to be mixed to a smooth paste, but check the manufacturer's instructions as the **amount of peroxide** will vary if you are using **liquid**, as opposed to **cream**, peroxide.

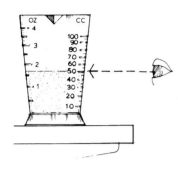

Powder bleaches are also strong bleaches and are generally used for highlights and fashion effects. However, they do have a tendency to **dry out** and become powdery if excessive heat is applied.

Always measure, check and mix bleach products carefully, checking the manufacturer's instructions. If you use peroxide that is too strong or mixtures of bleach that are too thick, you could burn the client's scalp and give an uneven colour to the hair. Peroxide that is too weak and bleach mixtures that are too thin can run into the client's eyes, skin and clothes and will not lighten the hair enough.

The chemistry of bleaching

All bleaches are **alkaline** and contain ammonia (you can smell this quite strongly when mixing bleaches).

The alkali in bleaches has two actions:

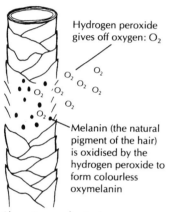

Hydrogen peroxide gives off oxygen: O₂

Melanin (the natural pigment of the hair) is oxidised by the hydrogen peroxide to form colourless oxymelanin

Changing melanin to oxymelanin

- it swells the hair and **opens up the cuticle** scales so that the bleach can enter the **cortex** and lighten the colour pigments
- it mixes with the hydrogen peroxide (releasing the acid stabiliser in the peroxide) and **releases the oxygen**, which will bleach out the colour.

Hair when bleached will always lighten in this order:

black
dark brown
medium red brown
light warm brown
light golden brown
medium golden blonde
light blonde
very light blonde
white (disintegration)

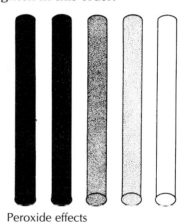

Peroxide effects

Hair must **never** be allowed to lighten beyond a very light blonde colour or it will disintegrate completely.

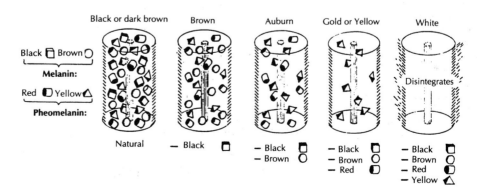

Bleaching out colour pigments

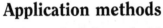

■ Take two test cuttings of naturally dark coloured hair. Bleach one of them with a little emulsion bleach, the other with a little powder bleach and 30 volume (9%) hydrogen peroxide, in a bowl.
■ Watch the development very carefully, wiping the bleach off every 10 minutes to see all the warm orange and yellow colours produced before the hair becomes blonde.

Application methods

Hair may be **lightened** with either highlift tint (mixed with special developers). emulsion bleach or powder bleach, depending on the **client's natural base shade** and the **degree of lift required**. Generally, dark hair will need the stronger bleach products to lift. If in any doubt, take a **test cutting**.

Whole head

Both whole-head and regrowth bleaches are usually applied to hair sectioned into four as shown in the diagram.

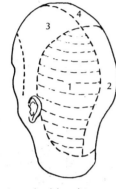

Sections for bleaching

Bleach is usually applied to the nape or crown area first where the hair is more resistant. Always apply bleach to a whole head of virgin hair in this order:

1. mid-lengths
2. ends of the hair
3. roots of the hair.

This is because the client's **body heat** (from the scalp) will make the bleach take **more quickly** near the scalp.

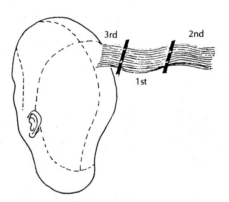

Whole-head bleach application

Never skimp with the amount of bleach. Take very small sections and always check the application thoroughly. The smallest area left uncovered will show up disastrously.

Regrowth application

When applying bleach to regrowth, you must always be thorough and **never overlap** on to the previously bleached hair, as hair breakage could occur.

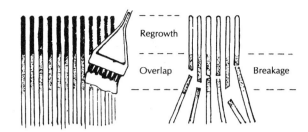

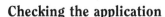

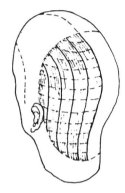

Hair breakage from overlapping

Cross-checking the application

Checking the application

You can never be too careful when applying bleach. Always check the application from the opposite direction to the one in which you applied it.

If you have missed any areas, apply bleach to them immediately, or dark patches will be seen. Pay special attention to the hairline and the thickest part of the hair (i.e. behind the ears).

Highlighting

Highlights also have the advantage that none of the product touches the scalp, which is useful for clients with sensitive scalps.

HEALTH MATTERS

When you are working in a strained position for a long time, as when doing cap or foil highlights, lower the height of the chair or ask the client if they can settle a little lower in the chair for you. These day-to-day strains can accumulate, becoming exhausting, and could result in permanent damage if care is not taken.

Try to keep your elbows down and close to your body whenever you can. Remember – keep a good posture at all times.

The cap method

Always brush the hair thoroughly before putting on the cap. This will ensure that the highlights show in the correct areas of hair.

Sometimes it is painful for the client when the highlight cap is put on, as it must be fixed securely and as close to the scalp as possible. A little talcum powder sprinkled inside the cap will make it easier to pull on.

Pull strands of hair through the cap using a highlight hook. Start pulling the strands through from the edges of the cap first to check the required thickness. This way, if the strands are too thick, they can easily be pulled back under the cap again with the highlight hook.

Once the strands have been pulled through, mix the bleach and then apply it thoroughly to all the hair strands. Check, then develop.

The advantage of this method is that it is very quick and easy.

Woven highlights

These are done with either foil or 'Easi-Meche' strips. Preparing woven highlights is a highly skilled technique.

Prepare the hair by sectioning in the 'nine-section' method (described in Chapter 5) so that you can work methodically, step by step.

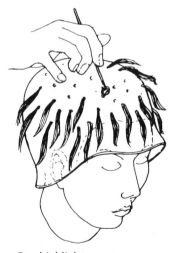

Cap highlights

Take sub-sections of hair of a similar size to those used for perming, and weave out the hair with a pin-tail comb. Place the woven strands on to the correct length of foil or Easi-Meche, apply bleach then re-seal the packets. Always start from the nape and work upwards.

When weaving out the strands of hair, always check that the strand directly below is woven, or the client will end up with stripes. As this is a lengthy process, some of the highlights may have developed to the required degree of lightness before completion, so check the development continually. If some highlights are ready, then stop the development on those strands only with cotton wool and warm water.

You might have to re-mix some fresh bleach if it takes you a long time (over 45 minutes) to complete the head, as the bleach mixture loses its strength after a time.

The advantages of woven highlights are that they are more comfortable for the client, you can see exactly where the highlights are being placed, you can mix tint and bleach highlights and the product can be applied closer to the root area than with the cap method.

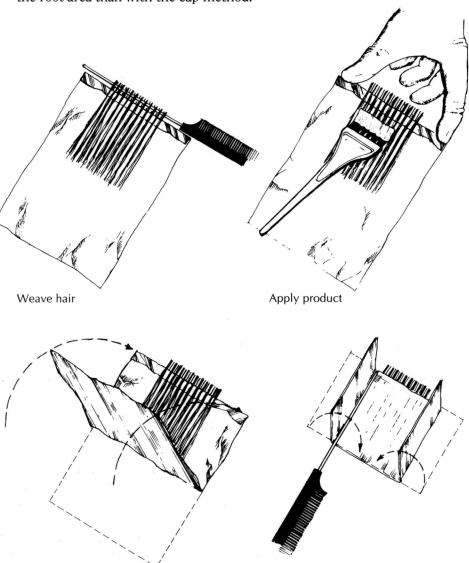

Weave hair   Apply product

Fold foil lengthways   Complete parcel

To do

- Practise woven highlights on models who can spare the time, using thick conditioning cream instead of bleach.

Lowlights

Lowlights are colours which are **darker** or **have more tone** (e.g. golden, warm, red or silver) than the **client's natural base** shade. These are applied in the same way as cap or woven highlights. Often two or three colours are used together for woven highlights to give many varied and natural effects. For instance gold, copper, and light red colours woven alternately on to a dark blonde base can look particularly good.

Clients who have a lot of white hair around the front hairline may prefer a colour that matches their base shade woven into the white hair. This will blend the colour in, and regrowth won't be so obvious when the hair grows out.

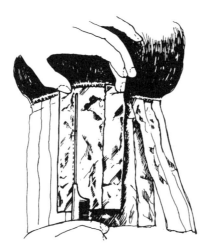

Bleach highlights with foil

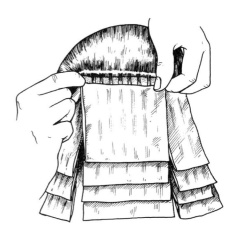

Tint lowlights with self-adhesive strips

Checking and timing the bleach

Remember

A **warm** salon will make the bleach take quicker. A **cold** salon will slow down the bleaching process.

Apart from checking that you have not missed any areas of hair with the bleach, always make sure that no bleach has **spilt on to the client's skin**. If it has, remove it immediately with a dampened piece of cotton wool.

Time the bleach according to the manufacturer's instructions, but remember to **test** at frequent intervals.

Testing

To test whether the bleach is ready, wipe the product from the hair with damp cotton wool and water. Then lay the strand over another piece of dry cotton wool so that you can see the true colour.

Hairdressers often do an **elasticity test** (sometimes called a **tensile strength** test) at this stage, using their fingers, to test the amount of elasticity in the hair.

To do

■ Re-read the section in Chapter 1 on elasticity tests and strand tests.

Removing the bleach

Whole-head or regrowth bleach
Remove the bleach product by rinsing thoroughly until the water runs clear. Use a lower water temperature than usual because the client's scalp will be sensitive, but ask the client if the temperature is comfortable.

Then **gently** shampoo the hair. If a bleach toner is to be used then do not use a conditioner, otherwise use an acid anti-oxy conditioner to return the hair to its natural acid state and close the cuticle scales.

Woven highlights
Carefully remove the tin foil or Meche from the hair, then proceed as for a whole-head or regrowth bleach (above).

Cap highlights
Rinse the bleach from the highlights then use either a little shampoo or conditioner. Gently ease off the cap then proceed as for a whole-head or regrowth bleach (above).

Complete the record card.

> **Remember**
>
> Bleaches always affect hair condition – the hair appears duller, more porous and more likely to break at the ends. Always recommend and use conditioners.

Test your knowledge

1 What is the difference between highlights and lowlights?
2 List all of the tools and equipment available for highlighting or lowlighting hair and how they are used
3 What effect does a warm salon have on the bleaching process?
4 How does the client's body heat affect bleach development?
5 Name two effects that hydrogen peroxide would have on hair if it were used by itself.
6 What is always released from hydrogen peroxide when it is mixed with bleaching products?
7 Which part of the hair is affected by bleach mixtures?
8 Why are bleaches always alkaline?
9 List the causes and corrections of the following problems
 ■ hair damage/breakage
 ■ skin/scalp damage
 ■ hair not light enough
 ■ hair over-lightened
 ■ uneven colour result.
10 What are your responsibilities to your client under the COSHH Act?
11 Why should you check with your supervisor if you are unsure about how to correct any mistakes?

Summary of bleaching faults and corrections

Always check with your supervisor that you have chosen the proper correction to match the fault beforehand

Fault	Causes	Corrections
Hair damage/breakage	Applying bleach (overlapping) on to previously bleached hair	Re-condition the hair and apply restructurants
	Incorrect proportions of mixture or too many boosters/activators used	
	Too high a concentration of hydrogen peroxide used	
	Over-developing the bleach, leaving it on too long (often due to not taking a strand test)	
	Processing with too much heat	
Skin/scalp damage	Not using barrier cream around the hairline	If just a little sore, then apply a soothing moisturising cream
	Use of too strong a bleach mixture	If very inflamed, seek medical attention
	Over-developing the bleach: leaving it on too long	
	Cuts and abrasions on the scalp before bleaching	
Hair not light enough	Client's base colour too dark for the strength of bleach mixture used	Test hair elasticity and porosity: if satisfactory then re-bleach
	Bleach mixture too weak: peroxide strength too low	Apply a silver, ash or matt toner (for yellow, orange or red hair tones)
	Insufficient development time: bleach not left on long enough	
Hair over-lightened	Use of too strong a bleach mixture	Re-condition the hair, apply restructurants
	Over-developing the bleach: leaving it on too long	Re-colour under supervision
Uneven colour result	Uneven application	Spot bleach darker areas and re-bleach if under-processed
	Overlapping	
	No allowance made for body heat on a whole-head application	
	Bleach mixed badly, lumps left in the mixture	
	Sections too large	
	Application too slow	
	Seepage of product out of foils/meche	

Temporary colours

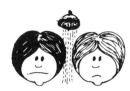

Temporary colours are very popular because they create an **instant** colour change. They are quick to apply and easy to remove if the client is dissatisfied with the result.

Temporary colours are useful for adding stronger **tones** to natural or artificially coloured light or dark hair, e.g. warm golden, ashen, rich auburn.

Sometimes natural white hair or bleached hair looks too yellow or golden (brassy) and benefits from being neutralised by silver tones.

However, blending in a few grey hairs (remember grey hair is white and naturally coloured hair mixed together) may be more difficult. Some colours produce unwanted warm (orange/red) overtones on white hair.

Temporary colours can also be used to darken natural and artificially coloured hair.

Remember
Temporary colours **wash out** of the hair the first time you shampoo.

To do
■ Use your temporary colour shade chart to match and select several different colours for different clients. ■ Check your choice with your supervisor. If you are a little unsure either take a test cutting (see Chapter 1) or try out a little of the colour on the underneath of the hair.

Make a note of the colour used on a record card.

Forms of temporary colours available and their application

Coloured mousse	Coloured setting lotion	Colour shampoos	Coloured hairspray
Apply to towel-dried hair: shake the container thoroughly, squeeze the nozzle, then apply to the palm of your (gloved) hand and spread over the hair with your fingertips	Apply to towel-dried hair: either sprinkle on the hair from the bottle, or (to even out colour on more porous hair) apply to small sections with a bowl and brush. These lotions also help to keep the set in place	These are shampooed onto the hair at the basin to enhance the hair colour. They are rinsed out and do not contain styling aids.	Spray on to dry hair after styling. Remember to protect other areas (such as the client's face) with tissue when spraying

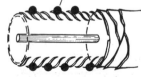

Colour molecule

The chemical action of temporary colours

The chemistry of temporary colours

The **pigment molecules** of temporary colours are **too large** to enter the hair shaft, so they coat the **outside** of the hair. This is why they are washed away so easily.

However, **unevenly porous** hair (e.g. permed and highlighted ends) will always **take a temporary colour unevenly**. The **cuticle scales** are swollen and **open in porous hair** and the large colour molecules can become trapped there and not wash out.

Test your knowledge

1 What types of temporary colours are available in the salon?
2 What colour tone would you recommend for a client whose blonde highlights are too yellow?
3 Name the part of the hair that is affected by temporary colour.
4 How long should a temporary colour last on the hair?
5 State how the client's natural hair colour depth and tone will affect the temporary colour result.
6 State the effect of applying a temporary hair colour to unevenly porous hair.

Semi-permanent colours

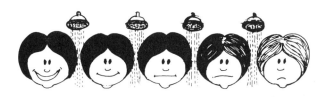

Semi-permanent colours have the advantage of colouring and conditioning hair at the same time. They do not need to be mixed with hydrogen peroxide and so do not leave any regrowth.

They are useful for blending in a small amount of white (grey) hair, but are not strong enough colours to cover a lot of white hair.

To do

■ Use your semi-permanent colour shade chart to match and select several different colours for different clients, including very light blonde, medium brown and very dark brown base shades.
■ Check your choice with your supervisor. If you are a little unsure about the result then take a test cutting (see Chapter 1) and show the result to your client.

Colour molecule

The chemistry of semi-permanent colours

The chemistry of semi-permanent colours

The pigment molecules of semi-permanent colours are **smaller** than those of temporary colours and so are able to penetrate a **little way into the cortex** of the hair. They tend to wash out slowly and so last longer than temporary colours.

Unevenly porous hair (e.g. permed, relaxed or bleached hair) will also take a semi permanent colour **unevenly**. The **cuticle scales are swollen** and **open in porous hair** and the smaller molecules can penetrate deeper into the cortex in the porous part of the hair, although they rinse off normally from the non-porous parts – **producing patchy results**.

Preparing the client

- Re-read the section on preparing the client for colouring or bleaching. Assess the amount of white hair present. Semi-permanents will cover only a small amount of white hair. Take a test cutting if you are unsure of the result.
- Pay special attention when gowning up for semi-permanent colours because they are **stain dyes**. They will stain your hands or your client's skin in the same way that a felt tip pen stains. So make sure you wear gloves and protect your client's skin with barrier cream.
- Some of the newer semi-permanents on the market now last up to 15 shampoos because they contain a stronger ingredient called **para**. If this is the case then the client must have a skin test (see Chapter 1). These colours are different because they are always **mixed with a low strength of hydrogen peroxide** and are known as **quasi**, or sometimes oxy-, permanents. They give a better coverage of white hair and an excellent shine, but can leave a slight regrowth.

To do

- Check the manufacturer's instructions on the semi-permanent colours in your salon to see if any of them need a skin test.

- Check the manufacturer's instructions before shampooing. You normally give one or two shampoos – but no conditioner – then towel dry the hair before applying the product.
- Also check the manufacturer's instructions for mixing. Some products are applied directly from the bottle, tube or flask while others are poured into a bowl and applied with a sponge or brush.

Application methods

- Use the correct amount of product for the length of hair (short hair needs less than long hair). Check with your supervisor if you are in doubt about how much to use.
- Mix or **prepare the colour** according to the manufacturer's instructions.
- **Divide the hair** into four large sub-sections and secure with section clips.
- Take neat, even partings for the sub-sections. Hair that is generally **thick** and products with a thick consistency need smaller sections, and vice-versa.
- Start working from the **crown downwards** and keep the hair controlled so that it does not fall on the client's skin.
- **Speed** is very important when applying semi-permanent colours as they do not take long to process or develop.
- When you have finished, **cross-check** the application (check by taking sections in the opposite direction from the way in which you applied it). Remove any skin staining with damp cotton wool immediately.

Developing and timing the colour

- Make sure that the hair is sufficiently **loosened** to allow the circulation of air.
- Check the hair colour development by taking a **strand test** (see Chapter 1). Remember that over-porous hair develops quickly.
- The development time will vary from 5 to 45 minutes, depending on the manufacturer, so check the instructions.

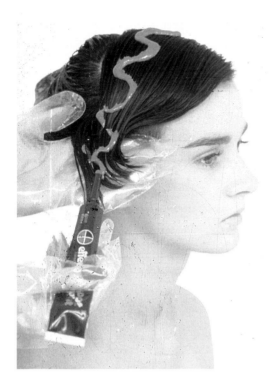

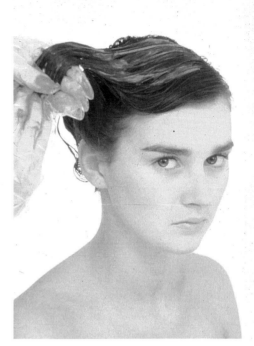

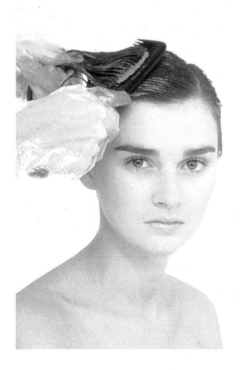

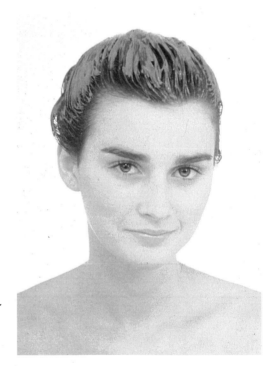

Removing the colour

Most semi-permanents are removed by thorough rinsing with warm water and lathering, as the hair has already been shampooed. (Always check the manufacturer's instructions to make sure).

Feel the hair to make sure it is clean and use a conditioner if needed. Complete the record card.

Summary of semi-permanent colour faults and corrections

Always check with your supervisor that you have chosen the proper correction to match the fault before attempting the correction.

Fault	Causes	Corrections
Incorrect colour result	Failure to show the client the shade chart while discussing the colour	Shampoo repeatedly until the colour has faded
	Incorrect analysis of hair (not noticing strong, porous or white hair)	
	Not taking a test cutting	
	Under or over-developing the colour	
Skin staining	Colour used on a very dry scalp	Remove with dampened cotton wool or skin stain remover
	Barrier cream not used around the client's hairline	
Patchy result	Poor application	Shampoo repeatedly until the colour has faded.
	Sections too large	
	Application not checked	If this does not work then try using either white spirit and cotton wool to dry hair or a **brightening shampoo** (equal parts 10 vol. peroxide and shampoo) or try a **bleach bath** (equal parts powder bleach/warm water and shampoo)
	Unevenly porous hair: has absorbed the colour unevenly and become patchy	

Test your knowledge

1 Why is gowning up especially important when using semi-permanent colour?
2 State how skin staining is best avoided when applying semi-permanent colours.
3 What is the average length of time a semi-permanent colour should last?
4 What is the difference between applying a semi-permanent colour and a temporary colour?
5 Which parts of the hair are affected by semi-permanent colours?
6 State how the client's natural hair colour depth and tone will affect the semi-permanent colour result.
7 State the effect of applying a semi-permanent colour to unevenly porous hair.
8 Describe two correction methods that may be used if the semi-permanent colour has produced uneven results.
9 What are your responsibilities to your client under the COSHH Act?
10 Why should you check with your supervisor if you are unsure about how to correct any mistakes?

Permanent colours

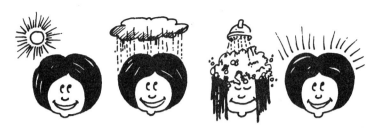

There are three main types of permanent hair colour.

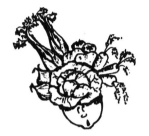

Natural vegetable dyes

The most common of these is **henna**, which gives copper or red tones to the hair. It works by coating the hair shaft and sticking to the outside cuticle layer.

Metallic dyes

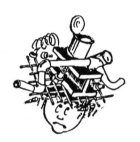

These are sold in shops as hair **colour restorers** (e.g. Grecian 2000). **Never perm**, **tint** or **bleach** over hair dyed with metallic dyes – it will break off. (Re-read the section in Chapter 1 on incompatibility tests).

Synthetic (man-made) dyes

Permanent tints are **para** dyes and are known as **oxidation** dyes because they are always mixed with hydrogen peroxide.

The widest possible choice of colours is available with permanent tints. They can be used to darken or lighten (up to four shades lighter), and have a whole range of subtle and vibrant tones (see the ICC chart on page 106).

(see the ICC chart on page 106)

> **Remember**
>
> Permanent colours **last until they grow out**. Regrowth tints need to be applied every 4–6 weeks.

To do
■ Use your permanent colour shade chart to match and select several different colours for different clients.
■ Check your choice with your supervisor.
■ If you are not quite sure about the result, take a test cutting (see Chapter 1) and show the result to your client.

Forms of tint available

Creams (tube)
These are mixed to a creamy consistency and are particularly good for covering coarse, resistant hair.

Oil-based tints (bottle)
These liquids mix to a gel-like thickness and give a more natural finished look.

Oil/cream emulsion (tube/bottle)
These have the benefits of both creams and gel tints and are easy to work with.

Mixing tints

All tints are mixed with hydrogen peroxide (either liquid or cream) and often in equal parts, e.g. 60 ml of tint and 60 ml of hydrogen peroxide.

Mix your tint just a few minutes before you need to use it – it will 'go off' if you mix it too soon.

To do

■ Look up the section on hydrogen peroxide earlier in this chapter to check the different uses for different strengths of peroxide (e.g. 10, 20, 30, 40 and 60 vol.).

The chemistry of permanent tints

Tints are alkaline so will swell the hair and **open up the cuticle scale**s, allowing the colour to **enter the cortex**.

All tints are made of small molecules of **para** dye mixed with hydrogen peroxide. These small molecules of tint **link** with the **hydrogen peroxide** inside the hair shaft to form larger molecules which cannot escape. This is called an **oxidation reaction**.

Once the colour has developed it remains permanently inside the hair shaft, and an **acid anti-oxy rinse** is applied after shampooing to close down the cuticle scales.

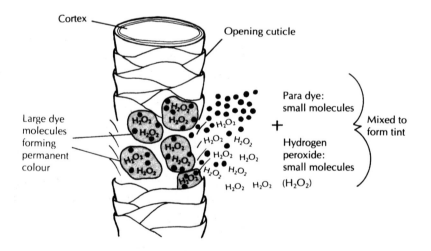

The chemistry of permanent colours

To do

■ Read the containers of permanent tints in your salon to see the ingredients and whether they contain the word **para.**

Preparing the client

- Re-read the section on preparing the client for colouring and bleaching (p. 110).
- Assess the amount of **white hair** present – remember, bright colours will show up stronger on white hair. Again, either check with your supervisor or take a test cutting if you are unsure.

- Do not **shampoo** before a tint unless the hair is excessively greasy or full of hairspray, when you should shampoo and dry the hair thoroughly. The only other exception is when you are going to apply bleach toners to towel-dried hair.
- Use the **correct amount** of tint. Half a tube is normally sufficient for a regrowth while a whole tube should normally be used for a (short) whole-head, very thick hair or comb-through application.
- Wear **gloves** to prevent dermatitis.

Application methods

Always divide the hair into equal sections (usually four).

Regrowth application

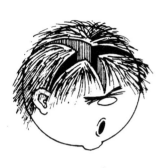

Take neat, even partings for the sub-sections. Thick hair and products with a thick consistency need smaller sections, and vice versa.

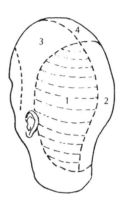

Apply the tint to the **roots**, starting at the back using 6 mm partings. However, if there is any resistant white hair at the front you should start in that area. **Do not overlap** with the previously tinted hair or the colour will be uneven and patchy. You need to work in a neat, speedy manner without spilling or splashing the tint.

To do
■ Practise applying a thick conditioning cream to a model's hair to the roots only and time yourself. It should not take more than 20 minutes.

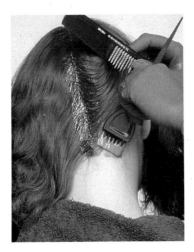

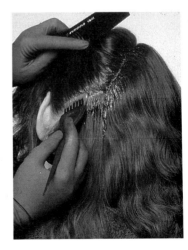

127

Summary of permanent tinting faults and corrections

Always check with your supervisor that you have chosen the proper correction to match the fault before you attempt the correction.

Fault	Causes	Corrections
Colour too light	Tint not left on long enough: under-processed Hydrogen peroxide too weak: colour molecules not developed properly Hydrogen peroxide too strong for the amount of tint required	Re-tint the hair using the correct strength of peroxide and developing for the correct length of time
Insufficient coverage	Strong coarse hair (often white) Peroxide strength weakened during process Make-up or barrier cream on the hairline	Pre-soften with 10 vol. peroxide then apply tint and peroxide mixed Re-apply with fresh tint and peroxide Clean with spirit and re-apply tint.
Colour too dark	Colour choice too dark Over-porous hair (perhaps from too many comb-throughs)	The hair can be lightened with either a colour reducer or a **softening** shampoo (a mix of 1 scoop powder bleach/30 ml 6% or 9% peroxide/60 ml warm water/15 ml shampoo); but this must be done by a senior member of staff
Patchy, uneven colour	Uneven application, overlapping, sections too large, insufficient tint used No allowance for body heat on a whole-head application Tint mixed badly, lumps left in the mixture Application too slow Unevenly porous hair	Correct by spot tinting to the lighter areas
Scalp irritated	Peroxide too strong Allergic reaction to tint	Immediately remove with cool water
Colour too ash (green)	Not prepigmenting (i.e. using a warm colour before applying the base shade when returning a bleached/lightened client to their natural colour) Chlorine from swimming pools	**Bleach bath** (a mix of equal parts powder bleach/ warm water/ shampoo) to cleanse and remove the ash tone
Colour too red	Colour choice too red Too much white hair present Natural warmth in the hair	Re-tint with a matt (green) colour of the same depth
Colour too orange	Colour choice too orange (copper) Too much white hair present Natural warmth in the hair	Re-tint with an ash (blue) colour of the same depth
Colour too yellow	Colour choice too golden Too much white hair present Natural warmth in the hair Peroxide too strong	Re-tint with a silver (violet) colour of the same depth

Check the application by sectioning in the opposite direction and re-applying to any uncovered areas.

If the ends are faded the colour may need to be combed through. This is not done every time as it damages the hair, making it more porous. Normally, diluted tint is applied to the ends for the **last few minutes** of the development time, and the hair massaged with the fingers to distribute the tint evenly.

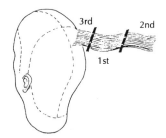

Whole-head application

For a whole-head application the tint it always applied to the **mid-lengths and ends**, then to the roots of the hair, unless the hair is very short. This is because heat from the client's scalp will make the tint take more quickly on the roots and speeds up the processing time.

Developing and timing the tint

- Make sure that the hair is sufficiently **loosened** to allow the circulation of air.
- Check the manufacturer's instructions to see **how long** it should be left before checking (the average time is 30 minutes), and whether you should use **heat** (from an accelerator), which will halve the development time.
- Check the colour development by taking a **strand test** (see Chapter 1). Remove some of the colour from the roots and the ends and compare the two colours. If they are of the required shade then remove the colour.

Removing the tint

Take the client to the wash-basin and add a small amount of **water** to loosen the colour whilst massaging the head. Rinse off the tint thoroughly with tepid water until the water runs clear. Use a cream or an **acid-balanced shampoo**, massage gently, then rinse. Apply a second shampoo if necessary.

Use an acid **anti-oxy conditioning rinse** to prevent the tint from oxidising any further and to close the cuticle scales. Complete the record card.

> **Remember**
>
> A **warm** salon will make the tint take quicker, a **cold** salon will make the tint take more slowly.

Colour reducers

Colour reducers or colour strippers are used to **remove permanent tints** from the hair instead of using bleach.

They may be mixed with either water or peroxide, according to the desired result. Always check the manufacturer's instructions for mixing, application method and development time as these vary from one manufacturer to another

Remember

Colour reducing is a very specialised process and uneven colour results can occur if reducers are incorrectly applied. It is best done by a senior member of staff.

The reducers work by breaking down the large dye molecules (which form tint colours permanently inside the cortex) into small dye molecules. These are then washed out of the hair after development time. This effectively reverses the dye process.

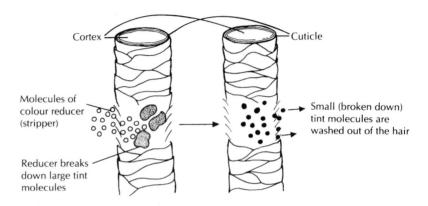

The chemistry of colour strippers

The colour does not always strip easily out of the hair and often leaves the hair an uneven colour. A second application of colour stripper is often necessary to achieve an even colour, and a tint should **always** be applied afterwards to achieve the final result.

Darkening bleached/lightened hair – prepigmentation

Prepigmentation or **colour filling** is a technique used to compensate for the **loss** of **yellow**, **orange** and **red** pigments from **bleached** or **lightened** porous hair.

If this is **not** done when returning bleached or lightened hair to the client's natural base colour the result will be **green** or ashen.

Prepigmentation chart

ICC Colour depths	Bleached colour tones	Prepigmentation colour tones needed
10: Lightest blonde	Very pale yellow	
9: Very light blonde	Pale yellow	Yellow (golden)
8: Light blonde	Yellow	Yellow (golden)
7: Blonde	Orange-yellow	$\frac{3}{4}$ Yellow (pale golden), $\frac{1}{4}$ orange (copper)
6: Dark blonde	Orange	$\frac{1}{2}$ Yellow (golden), $\frac{1}{2}$ orange (copper)
5: Light brown	Reddish orange	Orange (copper)
4: Brown	Reddish brown	Red
3: Dark brown	Brown	Red
2: Very dark brown	Dark brown	Red
1: Black	Black	Red

Remember

Bleached or lightened porous hair will develop quickly, so constantly check the development by taking a strand test using cotton wool. It may be ready **sooner than you expect.**

Always use a base shade **one shade lighter** than required. You can always add a darker colour later, but it is very difficult to remove dark colours from over-porous hair.

There are several techniques to choose from.

- Use a **semi-permanent** yellow, orange or red colour first. Shampoo the hair, towel dry it, apply the semi-permanent colour, develop it, then **blot off any excess** with cotton wool. Apply one shade lighter than the required base colour tint mixed with peroxide directly over the top of the semi-permanent colour. Develop as normal.
- Use a **permanent** yellow, orange or red tone first. **Do not** use any **peroxide**. Apply it to dry hair, then **blot off any excess** with cotton wool. Apply one shade lighter than the required base colour tint mixed with peroxide directly over the top. Develop as normal.
- Use a **permanent** tint and peroxide, one shade lighter than the required base colour with a strong yellow, orange or red tone. Develop as normal.

Safety points to remember when colouring or bleaching

- Always **read**, **check** and **follow** the manufacturer's instructions. Measure all colouring products accurately.
- Make sure you have completed any necessary **tests**, such as porosity tests, elasticity tests, incompatibility tests, skin tests or test cuttings before you start.
- Always **agree the final colour** with your client **before** starting.
- **Gown up** thoroughly so that no colour or bleach can stain the client's clothes.
- Apply **barrier cream** carefully to the client's hairline (but not their hair) before tinting or bleaching.
- Wear **rubber gloves** when applying all bleaches and colourants.
- If you spill any products, **clean up** immediately.
- Complete and file **record cards** immediately after use.

Test your knowledge

1 State how the client's natural hair colour depth and tone will affect the permanent colour result.
2 List the forms of tint available from various manufacturers.
3 Describe the effects of using different volumes of hydrogen peroxide for mixing with para tints.
4 What effect does a cold salon have on the tinting process?
5 How does body heat affect the application of a whole-head tint?
6 When would hydrogen peroxide be used by itself during tinting?
7 Which part of the hair is affected by para tints?
8 How do para tints work chemically on the hair?
9 How long should a permanent tint last on the hair?
10 Describe the effect of applying para tint to unevenly porous, highly sensitised hair (include any necessary precautions).
11 List the causes and corrections of the following problems
   - colour too light
   - colour too dark
   - insufficient coverage
   - patchy, uneven results
   - skin staining.
12 What are your responsibilities to your client under the COSHH Act?
13 Why should you check with your supervisor if you are unsure about how to correct any mistakes?

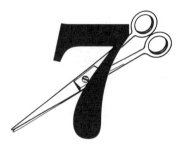

Reception

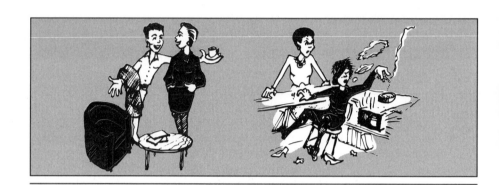

Remember

Reception is the most important area in the salon, because the clients visit reception first, and first impressions count.

The reception area not only attracts clients to the salon, but it is also where clients are greeted, appointments are made, the telephone is answered, bills are paid, records are kept, products are sold and clients are gowned up. The busy receptionist should look smart, be efficient and capable and always communicate pleasantly and politely with everyone who enters the salon.

The receptionist will have to:

- **greet** all clients and visitors with a smile and say 'Good morning/good afternoon, how may I help you?', then show them where to sit. Make sure the relevant person is informed that the client has arrived
- make all **appointments**
- answer the **telephone**
- **keep records** of salon services (perms, colours, etc.)
- use the **cash till** to take cash, cheques or credit card payments
- **sell products** displayed around the salon
- **explain** the services available to clients
- **gown up the clients** that are kept waiting (organise coffee, magazines, etc.)
- **receive deliveries** of stock
- **keep the reception area tidy** by always hanging up the clients' coats in the coat cupboard, removing any gowns left draped over chair, taking away any used coffee or tea cups, clearing the ash trays, tidying any piles of magazines, and always **making sure that no boxes or bags are left where someone could trip over them**
- help clients with their coats and **accompany them to the door**, checking whether they wish to make a further appointment and making sure that they have collected all their belongings
- be able to locate the **first-aid box**
- know where the **emergency exits** are, and understand the emergency procedures.

Remember

Not all salons have a receptionist, so you might have to carry out reception duties. Do it well: it is a very important job.

Tips for the receptionist

Always	Never
Look like a professional hairdresser: style your hair properly, wear the appropriate clothes and look after your hands and nails	Look untidy: forget to press your clothes, wear laddered tights, wear scuffed, down-trodden shoes, or forget to wear make-up
Act in a professional manner	Smoke, eat, drink or chew gum
Smile, and look at the client, paying attention to what you are doing	Look fed-up or bored or continue chatting with someone who works in your salon
Sit up properly	Slouch across the reception desk
Greet the client by name (you will know it from the appointment page)	Refer to the client as 'the 2.30'
Show the client where to sit	Make the client find their own seats
Apologise to the client if there is any delay	Keep clients waiting without explaining to them that there is a slight problem
Offer the client books, magazines, tea or coffee	Expect clients to help themselves
Deal with any problems in a positive way, e.g. 'I'm sorry, but the last client was a little late, so you may have a short wait'	Look flustered or become aggressive if there are problems. If you cannot deal with a problem, say 'Would you excuse me for a moment?' and fetch your supervisor

Making appointments

Remember

Many salons have a policy of never turning away a client, so always check with the stylists before offering an appointment at another time.

Remember

Appointments are always made in **pencil**, so they can be rubbed out if cancelled or changed.

Recording appointments

Expected clients, who have already made an appointment, may show you their appointment card or may have made the appointment on the telephone. In either case you need to check the client's name, time and service and the stylist's column on the appointment page. You can then pencil a tick by the client's name, and tell the stylist that the client has arrived.

You must record the same details on the appropriate page for **unexpected clients** – but you must check first that there is space available.

Always check the appointment details with the client.

Service abbreviations
These are the ones commonly used in the salon, but you may have others specific to some salons – if in doubt ask.

- C B/D – cut and blow dry
- S/S – shampoo and set
- P/W – permanent wave
- H/L – highlight
- L/L – lowlights
- B/D – blow dry

- C S/S – cut, shampoo and set
- T   – tint
- C/T   – conditioning treatment.

Some salons also write the client's telephone number just under their name. All of these services take different amounts of time. Here is a general guide:

- C B/D – short hair 30–45 minutes
- B/D   – short hair 15–30 minutes
         – long hair 30–45 minutes
- S/S   – 45 minutes to 1 hour
- P/W   – 2 hours + drying time
- H/L   – 1–1½ hours + drying time
- T   – 1 hour (regrowth only) + drying time.

Remember

Always allow time for longer processes to be completed, e.g. Gary's column: Mrs Smith P/W at 9.00 a.m. and B/D later (at 10.00 a.m.).

The appointment book

Here is an example of an appointment page. You can see here that more time must be allowed for longer processes such as perms and tints.

	SATURDAY, JULY 14th		
	GARY	DEBBIE	SHARON
0830	D. BROWN	G. TEBB H/L (foil)	M. HOWARD
0845	////// C B/D	/////////////	//////// C B/D
0900	MRS SMITH	//////////////	J. MOSSMAN
0915	/////// P/W	//////////////	/////// C B/D
0930	///////////////	D. SHAW	A.S. SMITH
0945	MRS JACOB S/S	//////// C B/D	/////// C B/D
1000	MRS SMITH B/D	G. TEBB	
1015	///////////////////	//////// B/D	
1030	MRS LOVELL Tint	F. SPENCER	
1045	/////////////////////	///// P/W (Restyle)	
1100	G. BRYANT	/////////////	
1115	/////// C B/D	/////////////	
1130	MRS LOVELL S/S	C. COATES	
1145	A. GREEN	/////// C B/D	
1200	//////// C B/D	F. SPENCER B/D	

Appointment cards

Most salons have appointment cards for clients to keep with the salon's name and telephone number and opening times printed on them. Once the client's appointment has been written in the appointment page, complete the appointment card with the date, day, service, time and stylist's name and then give the card to the client before they leave.

Salon price lists

These are often displayed at the reception area, but some salons also use printed cards. All the prices and services will be listed and it is a good idea for you to learn them.

Sometimes it is difficult to explain a certain price to a client. For instance, someone with long hair needing a cut and perm may be charged more than someone with short hair needing a perm but no cut. If in doubt call your supervisor.

Likewise, do not attempt to give long, elaborate explanations about the benefits of certain processes, such as multi-colour foil highlights, until you have been trained to do so. You could give the wrong information. Again, call your supervisor or one of the salon stylists.

Explaining the benefits

Every hairdressing service offered by your salon will benefit the client in certain ways. For example:

- a **permanent wave** gives more volume, bounce and lift to a hairstyle
- a **haircut** provides the foundations of a new hairstyle and removes split and damaged ends
- **highlights** give hair a lighter, brighter appearance, lifting the client's normal hair colour
- a **conditioning treatment** restores life to damaged, dry ends, giving shine and manageability.

To do
■ Make a list of each service offered by your salon and explain the benefits of each one.
■ Check the answers with your supervisor.

Using the telephone at reception

Remember

First impressions count. You are representing your salon – not chatting as you would to friends at home.

When you answer the telephone at reception, you must sound **professional**, **courteous**, and **friendly**. For instance, 'Hello, this is Headshape, how may I help you?' sounds much better than 'Yeah?'. You must always identify yourself or your salon and then find out who is calling and what they want to know.

Always replace the receiver carefully after receiving or making a call – otherwise your salon will be unable to receive any more calls, and business will be lost.

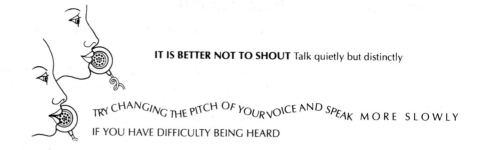

IT IS BETTER NOT TO SHOUT Talk quietly but distinctly

TRY CHANGING THE PITCH OF YOUR VOICE AND SPEAK MORE SLOWLY

IF YOU HAVE DIFFICULTY BEING HEARD

Tips for using the telephone

If you are cut off, replace the receiver and wait for the caller to ring again.

Always speak clearly.

Here are some ideas for making sure that you take down the correct letters and numbers when you are writing out information.

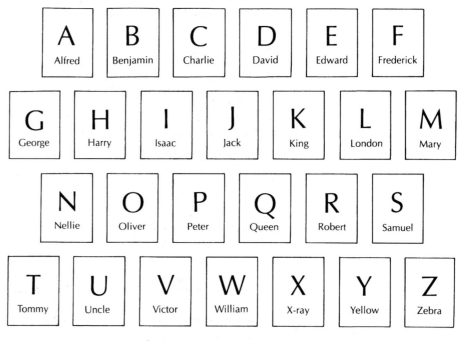

The telephone alphabet

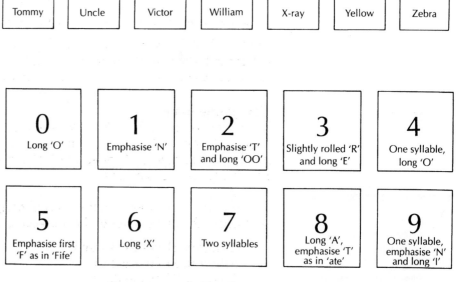

Number pronunciation

136

TELEPHONE MESSAGE PAD

From ... *Mr Green* ... Date .. *17/11*.
To *Caroline* .... Time .. *2.30pm*
Caller's Telephone No. .... *012578* ...

Message

Please call regarding his stock delivery of the new perm lotions.

Example of a message taken

Receiving calls

Here are some examples of the reasons people may have for calling your salon:

- to make, change or cancel an **appointment**. Always repeat the message to the person, e.g. 'Thank you that's Mrs Green, for a perm on Tuesday 2nd April at 1.00 p.m. We look forward to seeing you then'
- to make enquiries about **services**, e.g. cuts, perms, colours and their costs
- new clients may call to ask for the **salon location** and information on where to park their car
- people may call about **job availability** (you may need to check this with your supervisor)
- hairdressing company representatives (reps) may call to check on an order or to make an appointment to discuss **products** or equipment
- someone may make a **private call** to a member of staff. Check the salon policy about this, as some salons will allow emergency calls only and you might have to take message. (There is a sensible reason for this: potential clients cannot make appointments if the line is always busy.) Remember to **give the message to the relevant person** at an appropriate time. Some messages are confidential, so keep them in a safe place.

Making calls

There are three main telephone directories:

- *The phone book* (residential and business – listed alphabetically)
- *Yellow Pages* (business – listed by category)
- *The Thomson Directory* (local business – listed by category).

There are three main types of dialling code:

- local codes (you do not need to use one if you are making a call within your local area).
- national codes, e.g. London is 0181 or 0171
- international codes, e.g. 00 is used before dialling the country code for places outside the UK.

The phone book

You may have to use *The phone book* to find the telephone numbers of clients who do not have record cards at your salon. People are listed in *The phone book* in strict alphabetical order from A to Z: but remember, some people choose not to be listed.

You will find the entries set out in the following order: the surname or business name, the initial letter of the first name, then the address. For example:

> Abbott A, 21 Roydon Close
> Abbott B, 87 Ambrose Ct
> Abbott C, 29 Maine Road.

Yellow Pages

Yellow Pages is a directory for business use. For instance, if you need a plumber or an electrician, or if you want to find out where all the other hairdressing salons in your area are, you will find them listed alphabetically by category here.

There is a *Yellow Pages* for every county. The boundaries of the area covered by each *Yellow Pages* are shown on a map at the front of the book. There is also a list (or index) of categories at the front describing the type of service (e.g. hairdressers) or the goods supplied by the company (e.g. hairdressing suppliers or wholesalers).

Operator and telephone engineer services

Dial 100

This operator will help you if you have **difficulty in making a call** (for instance if the line is continually engaged and you have tried several times) or if your require special call services, such as transferred (reverse) charge calls or freephone calls.

Dial 192

This operator will help in finding any UK **number or dialling code**.

Dial 154

This will put you through to an engineer who deals with **faulty lines**. Tell them your telephone number and the nature of the fault.

999 calls: emergencies

If an accident happens you should call for assistance immediately.

- Lift the telephone handset and call the operator by dialling 999.
- When the operator answers, tell them the emergency service you want and your telephone number.
- Wait until the emergency authority comes on the line.
- Give the full address of where the emergency help is needed and any important and relevant information.
- Replace the handset.

Never make a **false call**. It is illegal, and you may be blocking the line for someone who urgently needs the emergency services.

Taking payments in the salon

Calculating the client's bill (including VAT)

Client's bills are written on a bill pad or a receipt slip, and usually torn off and given to the client to be checked before payment is made.

Remember

■ If you are **unsure of the correct price** to charge
■ If you find that the client's cheque, cheque card or credit card is **invalid** (out of date, or the signature does not correspond with the one on the cheque)
■ If the client **queries the bill**

Politely ask the client to wait for a moment, then **check the problem with your supervisor**.

To do

Watch a senior person in the salon working at reception when they are:

■ working the cash till
■ calculating a client's bill
■ taking money from a client and giving change
■ recording any products (e.g. hair spray) sold at reception.

A typical bill might look like the one below.

Date _____	
Client's name _____	
Stylist's name _____	
Service	Price
Cutting	☐
Blow drying	☐
Setting	☐
Permanent waving	☐
Conditioning treatment	☐
Colouring	☐
Bleaching/highlighting	☐
Other services, e.g. manicure	☐
Retail products	_____
Total	_____
(If applicable VAT is charged at 17.5% of the total cost) (+ VAT)	_____
Final total	_____

Many hairdressing businesses have to charge VAT (Value Added Tax) because they are supplying goods and services and exceed a certain income. This tax is then paid to the government at a later date. Some salons include VAT in the price, others add up the bill and then add on the VAT afterwards.

Vouchers

Some salons have special offers, gift vouchers or tokens which may be used instead of other forms of payment. Ask your supervisor if these are acceptable to your salon.

Cash payments

The cash till
Cash tills may be electronic or computerised. All tills will have:

- a container for cash or cheques
- a facility for recording the amount taken
- a facility for giving out a receipt.

Giving change
If you always follow the same procedure when giving change you are less likely to make mistakes. If your salon does not have a system you could follow this basic routine:

1. total the client's bill and tell them the cost
2. keep the money the client gives you on the till shelf (do not put the money straight into the till)
3. count out the change into your own hand
4. count the change into the client's hand and state how much you are giving
5. when the client is satisfied that the change is correct, put the money they gave you into the till
6. thank the client and give them the till receipt.

Payment by cheque

If the client is paying by cheque, make sure that it has been completed correctly. If it is not valid your salon will lose that money.

Follow this procedure:

1. make sure the client has a **cheque guarantee card** and accept it only if the expiry date (the month and year) has not passed
2. check that all the **words and figures** are entered correctly on the cheque
3. if the client has made a mistake, make sure that they have **initialed** the correction
4. check that the **account numbers** on the cheque card and the cheque (the last group of numbers on the bottom right hand side of the cheque) are the **same**, and that the **signature** on the cheque card matches the one on the cheque
5. write the cheque card number on the back of the cheque, then give the client their card and receipt.

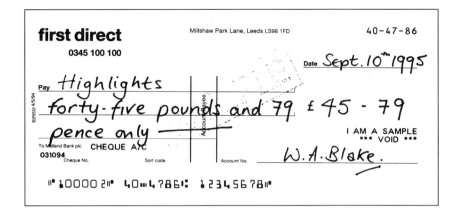

A correctly completed cheque

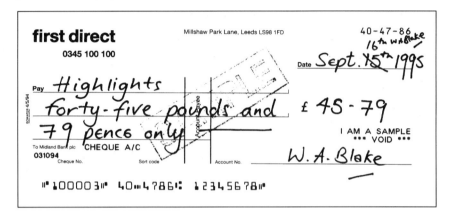

An initialled cheque

Payment cards

If your salon accepts payment cards (Access, Visa and Switch are the most common ones) a sticker will probably be displayed by the door or by the reception desk.

Follow this procedure:

1. first check that the payment card is **valid** (that the expiry date has not passed)
2. **complete the voucher** by writing in:
   - the date
   - the hairdressing service (e.g. 'perm', 'cut', or 'blow dry')
   - the amount to be charged

   Always use a ball-point pen, so that the writing can be seen on all three (carbon) copies

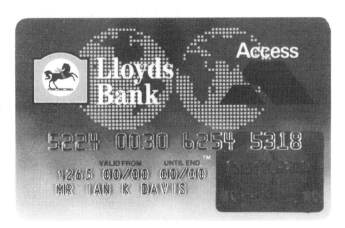

A credit card

3. place the card on the **imprinter** underneath the voucher, and press down the handle or slide it across so that the imprinter presses the numbers of the card and the name and address of the business on to the voucher
4. ask the client to sign the voucher in ball-point pen, then **check that their signature matches the one on the card**
5. give the client the **top copy** of the voucher as a receipt
6. **store** the other two copies of the voucher safely (perhaps in the cash till); one is kept for the salon, the other will be sent to the card company.

Cards can also be processed on automated machines that debit the account directly, so that only valid cards can be used. You should pass the card through the machine, then wait until it signals that the card has been cleared and types out the receipt. Ask the cardholder to sign the receipt and then check that the signature matches the one on the card. This is the only check that needs to be done when using this type of equipment.

To do

Watch a senior person working at reception when they are:

■ taking a cheque payment
■ taking a card payment.

Test your knowledge

(Re-read the sections in Chapter 1 on client care and communicating effectively with clients.)

1 List three reasons why it is important to communicate well with your client at reception.
2 Name two occasions when you should ask for help from your supervisor whilst attending to visitors and enquiries.
3 List your salon's procedure for taking messages.
4 Messages and record cards are confidential. Give two reasons why this is important.
5 List each of your salon's services and include the cost and time needed for each one.
6 Briefly describe your salon's appointment system, and include:
   ■ the procedures for dealing with expected and unexpected clients
   ■ service abbreviations
   ■ the timing of appointments
   ■ how you should communicate with the member of staff responsible for the scheduled service
   ■ how to take telephone calls and appointments
   ■ the information needed on an appointment card.
7 Where is your salon's list of retail products and prices located?
8 Describe the forms of payment that your salon accepts, include the details of an invalid payment and the procedure for dealing with a fraudulent payment.
9 Describe the ways you should deal with payment by cash, cheque and credit card.
10 Name two consequences of failing to handle payments correctly.
11 Name two consequences of failing to follow salon security procedures.

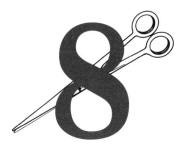

Working as a team

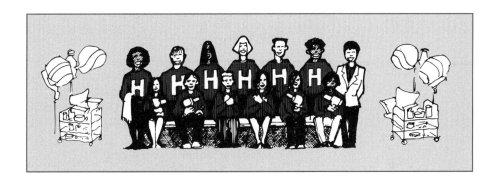

Who are the team members in a salon? They could be:

- other trainees
- junior and senior stylists
- supervisors
- managers
- others working in the salon such as receptionists, beauty therapists, people on work experience, cleaning staff or catering staff.

Salons vary in size – there might be just you and your supervisor in a small salon, you could be part of a medium-to-large salon of 4–20 people or part of a large chain of salons employing hundreds of hairdressers. Wherever you work, you will need to **do your own work well**, and **help and support the rest of the team** in an enthusiastic and pleasant manner.

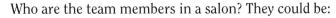

Good staff communication

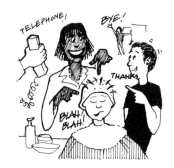

Remember
Look for any tidying or cleaning up that needs to be done in the salon – don't think that it is someone else's job!   Once that is done, stand and watch others at work – you should never stop learning in hairdressing.

Remember
Treat clients as you would like to be treated yourself.

Many clients return to a salon because it has a **good atmosphere** and the staff are always happy and cheerful. Tension or bad atmospheres in the salon can result in lost clients and poor working relationships.

- If someone asks you to help them always respond with a smile.
- If you need help yourself, ask for it as politely as you can, even if the pressure is on!
- Look and see who needs help in the salon and try to offer support (e.g. passing up perm papers) without being asked first.
- Don't offer to take on work without checking with your supervisor first (*you* may think you can attempt a new haircut, but does your *supervisor* think you can do it?)

Doing your own work well

Here is an example of a technical services checklist. It includes:

- what work you do
- when you did the work
- how you did the work
- where you did the work.

Technical Services – checklist

Your name ....

Type of service – tick   √
Cutting	Permanent Waving
Drying	Straightening
Dressing Hair	Colouring
Setting	Bleaching

Information required from stylist
MAKE AND TYPE OF LOTION
SIZES OF PERM RODS
WHICH WORKSTATION WILL BE USED

Information required from reception
TIME OF CLIENT ARRIVAL
RECORD CARD

List: Equipment needed	**List: Materials/products needed**
PERM TROLLEY	ACID P/W LOTION STRENGTH
GREY, BLUE, RED, P/W RODS	PRE-PERM LOTION
END PAPERS	WATER SPRAY
PLASTIC CAP	MANUFACTURERS INSTRUCTIONS
COTTON WOOL STRIPS	
BARRIER CREAM	
SECTION CLIPS	
PERM GOWNS AND TOWELS	
GLOVES	

Health and safety notes
CLIENT PROTECTION – GOWNS, TOWELS, COTTON WOOL, BARRIER CREAM
STYLIST PROTECTION – GLOVES
MANUFACTURERS INSTRUCTIONS, RECORD CARD FOR SPECIAL NOTES
SALON SAFETY – ALL WORK AREAS ARE LEFT CLEAN AND TIDY, AFTER THE
EQUIPMENT AND MATERIALS HAVE BEEN PUT AWAY. ANY CHEMICAL SPILLAGES ARE
MOPPED UP AND REMOVED

To do

Draw up similar checklists for yourself and complete one for each technical service.

Problems can happen

However well you prepare for the clients, problems can happen! For example:

- clients may be **late for appointments** (the bus was late, the car park was full)
- clients may arrive **without an appointment** (regular clients who have suddenly been invited out)
- a new receptionist could have **overbooked** (two Mrs Greens may turn up for the same appointment)
- a **service took longer** than the time allowed (the client may have had a complete re-style with their perm)
- the client may have **changed their requirement** (perhaps the stylist suggested a semi-permanent colour during client consultation for a haircut and it was added to that service)
- a **member of staff is suddenly absent** due to illness (remember to refer this immediately to your supervisor so that bookings can be rescheduled).

Resolving the problems

If there is a problem with the bookings, **keep cool, calm and don't appear flustered**! Politely ask the client to take a seat while you explain the situation to your supervisor. Your supervisor may suggest an alternative stylist, another appointment or a short wait.

If it is your job to look after the client until their appointment is started, **use your initiative**. Here are some suggestions of how to use the time:

- **explain the delay** to the client, giving an indication of how long they may have to wait
- **offer** the client **style books, magazines or newspapers** to read
- **offer** the client **tea, coffee or a soft drink**
- if the client is not having a chemical treatment, ask the stylist if you may **shampoo** the client and incorporate **a soothing scalp massage** (which should take up some of the waiting time)
- if the client refuses to wait and **cannot spare the extra time, tell your supervisor immediately**, don't wait until the client has left the salon!

Getting better at your job

You will need to identify your strengths and weaknesses within your role at work before you can improve yourself.

Strengths: what are you good at?

- Is it shampooing, cutting, perming, or colouring, for instance?
- Or are client relationships your strength?

Weaknesses: what are your weak points?

- Do you need to improve your technical services?
- Could you improve your speed?
- Could your relationships with the rest of the staff be improved?

To do

Make a list of your strengths and weaknesses and check them with your supervisor.

Reviews and feedback

Prepare yourself for a few negative comments from others. It is great to be told that you are better than you thought you were, but sometimes you may not be doing your best. **Always accept criticism in a positive manner** – remember you are still a trainee, and have much to learn.

Your supervisor may ask you to agree a target, which may mean, for instance, that in three month's time you will be able to wind a perm perfectly in 45 minutes. It will then be up to you to do enough practice to achieve that target. If you feel that perming is not your strong point, then you could ask for the target date to be set four or five months ahead.

Developments in technology

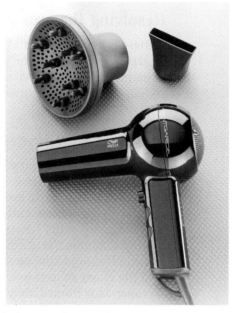

Remember

Be prepared: it is better to be practised and competent with new products and materials than to turn clients away.

Hairdressing is a fashion industry that is constantly changing, and to be able to create all the latest styles you must be able to use the most up-to-date tools and equipment and the most recently launched products.

Training courses/seminars

A **training course** generally consists of a trainer demonstrating new techniques and/or products, and then you having the opportunity to put them into practice.

A **seminar** consists of a similar demonstration, but for many more people.

Both training courses and seminars can be done 'in-house' – at the salon – or outside at a local college/training centre/manufacturer's training school or other suitable venue. To find out when training courses are available ask your supervisor or look up the trade journals such as *The Hairdressers Journal* or *The Cutting Edge*.

Test your knowledge

1 Describe three methods of effectively communicating in the salon that promote harmony within the team

2 In what circumstances would you check with your supervisor before starting a task?

3 List all the equipment and materials or products needed for the following technical services:
- cutting
- drying
- dressing hair
- setting
- permanent waving
- straightening
- colouring
- bleaching.

4 Describe the problems that could happen with client bookings and how you would resolve them.

5 In what circumstances would you check with your supervisor for rescheduled bookings?

6 Describe how you could use your time most productively if the salon was not busy.

7 Give two examples of what could happen if you forgot to pass on information to the salon team.

8 Describe your strengths and weaknesses for both technical and communication skills.

9 Why is it important to react positively to reviews and feedback from your supervisor?

10 List all the methods by which you could update your hairdressing knowledge.

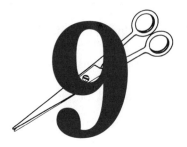

Salon resources

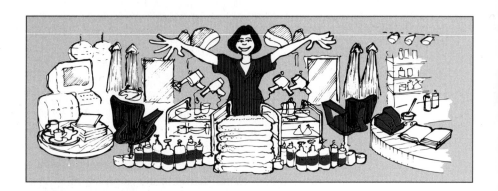

A hairdressing salon has many resources.

Stock

The stock is mostly hairdressing products, which may be:

- for **professional use** by the salon staff
- for **retail sales** to clients.

Fixtures and fittings

Examples of fixtures and fittings are the chairs, the dressing positions (or workstations), the wash-basins, the light fittings and the reception desk.

Utilities

- Power – the electricity supply
- Water – hot and cold
- Communication systems – telephones, intercom systems, computers, music systems.

Tools and equipment

This includes hair dryers, accelerators, scissors, clippers, razors, combs, brushes, tinting equipment, perming equipment, and trolleys.

Time

You are paid for your time *at work*, not just to work on a client's hair and to sit down doing nothing between clients. The salon must be kept clean, tidy and well stocked.

Space

Salon space should never be wasted. For instance a new delivery of stock must not be left by a stylist's workstation. It should be put into the storeroom immediately so that the workstation is free.

Salon resources are expensive

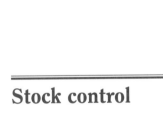

- Use resources for **approved purposes only** – e.g. don't use the salon telephone to chat to all your friends.
- Try to **minimise wastage** of stock, utilities, time and space e.g. turn off the lights when not in use, carefully measure out the amount of perm lotion or tint needed for each client.
- Make sure you know the **security procedures** for everything in your salon. In particular, don't leave keys in locks or lying around in the salon and don't leave valuables or products unattended.
- **Take care not to damage anything** in the salon – hairdressing salons are very expensive to equip. If you are not sure how to use something, ask for help.
- If you have any **ideas about improvements** in the salon – perhaps you have noticed that an electrical wire is worn and the wires are exposed – **tell your supervisor immediately.**

To do

- ■ Make a list of things that are sometimes wasted in the salon, then suggest one way wastage could be minimised.
- ■ Look around your salon and note which areas or equipment are the most damaged or worn. Think of three improvements that could help prevent wear and tear. Check your results with your supervisor.

Stock control

Hairdressing salons cannot run successfully without the correct amount and range of products or **stock**. However, stock is very expensive and old, unused stock remaining on the shelves wastes money. Existing stock must always be used before new packages are opened to **prevent wastage**. Using stock in **rotation** like this is called 'stock turnover'.

Types of stock

Stock for professional use, e.g. perms, relaxers, tints and colours, bleaches, shampoos and conditioners, neutralisers, styling products is usually kept in a stock room or a dispensary. Some of the styling products, shampoos and conditioners are kept available for instant use in the salon.

Stock for retail use, e.g. products and sundries (such as brushes, combs, hairdryers, hair ornaments, wigs or hairpieces) are sold to clients and the general public.

General stock also includes cleaning products and materials, personal protective equipment such as gowns, towels, protective capes, cotton wool, aprons and rubber gloves and sundries such as tea, coffee, milk and sugar.

149

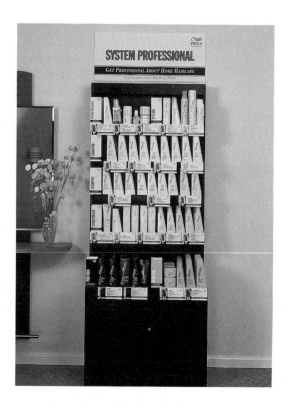

Remember

You cannot perm a client's hair if the salon has no perm lotion!

Always **immediately report any discrepancies** – shortages or surpluses – between the stock levels and the salon's records to your supervisor.

Remember

Always keep packages the right way up. Anything inadvertently placed upside down may leak or spill.

Recording stock

Your salon will have a specified method of recording stock levels for salon and retail use.

Stock records may be kept on anything from a notepad or book to a computer.

The following information is normally recorded:

- the date the stock is received
- the name of the supplier
- the quantity and type of stock received
- the value of the order.

Stock records must be checked regularly – this is called **stocktaking**. Stocktaking is done not only to see what needs to be re-ordered, but also to check which products (or sundries) are selling quickly or slowly.

When you are checking the stock against the records make sure that what you write is clear, legible, accurate and complete, as it will be checked again by your supervisor.

Stock that has been used is usually checked against the appointment book and the till receipt, giving a double record of where and when it was used. It may be your job to enter the stock delivery in the first place – if you make a mistake there may be problems at a later date if stock was found to be missing.

Stock deliveries

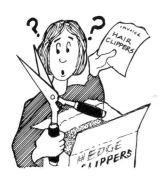

When new stock arrives at your salon:

- **unpack it very carefully** to avoid damaging the contents. If you are not sure how to open a package properly ask your supervisor
- immediately **remove any packaging materials** to avoid accidents or untidiness, but check with your supervisor as to how surplus packaging should be disposed of. It may be used for recycling and not just thrown in the bin!
- **check the stock for any damage** – this could include crushed boxes, broken lids, or labels peeling off
- **look at the sell-by dates** – your salon would not want to receive out-of-date stock!
- **report any damaged stock** immediately to your supervisor, who will deal with the problem and may be able to have the stock replaced
- make sure that the **contents match the delivery note**
- ask your supervisor if you may **check the delivery note** against the **original order**
- enter the details of the new stock correctly and accurately into your salon records (often a stock book)
- take the stock to the appropriate place for storage. Remember that all stock must be rotated, which means that old stock must be placed at the front of the storage space and new stock either placed behind it or kept for use at a later date. Products deteriorate after a period of time and will not work properly (e.g. opened bottles of liquid tint become oxidised by the air and will not colour hair successfully).

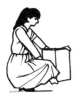

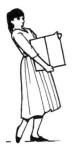

Always lift heavy loads with knees bent and back straight

To do

Read the section in Chapter 10 regarding the COSHH Act 1989: Storing and Using Salon Chemicals Safely.

Displaying stock for retailing

Many manufacturers supply special stands for displaying retail stock such as styling products, shampoos and conditioners for home use. As products are sold they should be replaced. You may be asked to restock the stands and to price the products.

- Stock must be **displayed safely** so that it cannot accidentally fall on anyone (hairdryers are particularly heavy) and out of the reach of children.
- Stock must be displayed in a **safe environment** at or below room temperature, away from naked flames and sources of heat – particularly direct sunlight. Many products, especially hairspray and nail polish remover, are highly flammable.
- Always check with your supervisor that the product is **correctly priced**.

New stock may be more expensive than older packages of the same product, or the salon may have a promotion or a 'special offer' and be selling stock at a lower price. If you have to stick new price labels on products make sure the label is clearly visible and does not cover over the name or the contents.

There are two types of retail goods:

- those with a **limited life** that have a sell-by date (e.g. shampoos, conditioners, and styling products). Remember to keep existing stock at the front and place new stock behind it
- products **without a limited shelf life** (e.g. brushes, combs, hairdryers. hair ornaments, wigs and hairpieces) also need to be sold in rotation in case they go out of fashion.

Test your knowledge

1 Describe your salon's procedure for stocktaking.
2 Why is it important to identify any shortages or surpluses of stock?
3 Why should stock be rotated?
4 Why should stock be displayed properly?
5 List the important points regarding the storage and display of stock relevant to the COSHH Act.
6 Why is it important to use salon resources only for approved purposes?
7 Describe how you could minimise wastage and damage in your salon.
8 Describe the possible consequences of failing to follow your salon's security procedures.

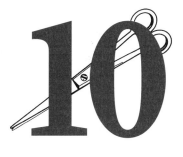

10 Health and safety in the salon

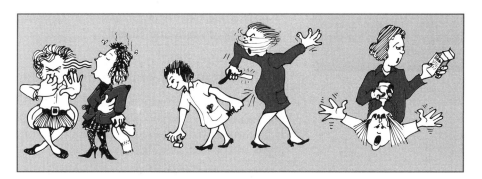

Hairdressers must always work:

- **Cleanly**. Both your client's health and your health is at risk. Tools and equipment must be clean and properly sterilised. There are many diseases that you and your client could catch from dirty equipment – such as head lice, impetigo and ringworm.
- **Safely**. Careless work could lead to hair loss, hair breakage, damage to the client's skin or eyes, or ruined clothes.

Did you know that legally you (the employee) must take care not only of your own health and safety, but also that of anyone else who may be affected by your work?

This means that you should:

- know where the emergency exists are in case of a fire or bomb alert
- know how to telephone for the emergency services (e.g. the fire brigade, the ambulance service)
- know which chemicals used in the salon are dangerous and how to use them safely
- know how to use electrical equipment safely
- have some knowledge of emergency first aid.

> **Remember**
>
> Accidents **can** and **do** happen. Be prepared.

Salon hygiene

Preventing the spread of infection

- Each hairdresser should have at least **two sets of tools**, one in use and the other being sterilised or disinfected ready for the next client.
- **Clean towels and gowns** should be given to each client. Towels should be **washed** and dried after use (not simply dried).

153

- **Hair should be swept up** after every haircut and placed in a covered container.
- All **work surfaces** must be **regularly cleaned** with hot water and detergent. Surfaces should be made of materials that are free of cracks and are easy to keep clean.
- Clients with any **infectious conditions** (e.g. head lice, ringworm or impetigo) **should not be treated in the salon** but tactfully referred to a doctor. If work begins before the problem is noticed, then the service should be completed as quickly as possible. Contaminated hair (e.g. hair with nits or head lice in it) should be swept up immediately and preferably burnt – if not, it should be placed in a sealed container. Hairdressing equipment and clothing that has been in contact with the client must be sterilised or disinfected.
- Care should be taken when using **tools which may cut** or pierce the skin or in areas with open, bleeding or weeping wounds or cuts because of the risk of AIDS and Hepatitis B.

Remember

If you accidentally drop any tools on the floor, **clean**, **dry** and **sterilise** them before using them on the next client. Broken tools must not be used because they can be a source of infection.

AIDS (Acquired Immune Deficiency Syndrome)

This is caused by a virus which attacks the natural defence system of the body so that the person is unable to fight a disease, and can lead to death. It is transmitted by blood or tissue fluid from an infected person entering a break in the skin of a healthy person.

Hepatitis B

This is a virus which attacks the liver. Hepatitis is a very serious disease, which can kill. It is transmitted by infected blood or tissue fluid coming into contact with the body fluids of an uninfected person, usually through a cut. Therefore combs, brushes, etc. should not be used on broken skin affected with boils or skin rashes (such as impetigo) unless they can be sterilised immediately afterwards. If you accidentally cut the skin with scissors, clippers or razors, these must immediately be cleaned and sterilised.

Sterilisation and disinfection

All tools such as brushes, combs and hair rollers must be thoroughly **cleaned** with hot soapy water to remove loose hairs, dust and dirt. Scissors and razors can be cleaned with alcohol. This must be done **before** sterilisation or disinfection.

Sterilisation
This means the killing of all organisms, whether

- fungi, e.g. ringworm
- bacteria, e.g. impetigo
- parasites, e.g. head lice.

Autoclaves
These are highly recommended, as they are the most efficient method for sterilising metal tools, combs and plastics (check beforehand that tools can withstand the heat). Autoclaves sterilise by the creation of **steam heat** (121°C) and **pressure**, and take about 20 minutes to work.

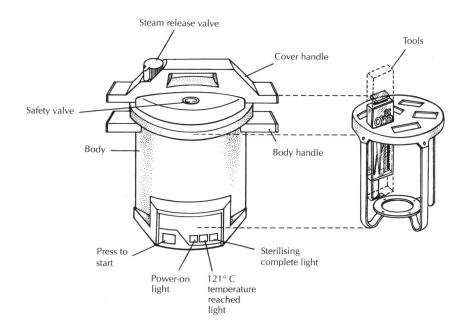

An autoclave

Boiling in water

Towels and gowns should be washed in a hot wash cycle, where the water should reach 95°C.

Ultraviolet radiation cabinet

These are used in many salons, but all the tools must be perfectly clean before being placed in this cabinet. During the process tools must be turned over frequently to expose all surfaces to the ultraviolet rays, which come from a mercury vapour lamp at the top of the cabinet. Each side of the tools should be exposed to the ultraviolet rays for 20–30 minutes.

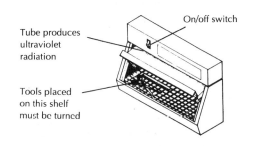

An ultraviolet cabinet

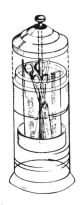

A disinfecting jar

Disinfectants

These chemicals are effective only they are if used correctly. They quickly become stale or overloaded, and must be used at the **correct concentrations** for the correct length of time.

Personal hygiene and appearance

Salon hygiene is extremely important – but personal hygiene is just as obvious to and necessary for your client.

Think how close you stand to clients when you are doing their hair. Both bad breath and body odour can offend, so keep your breath fresh and remember that soap and water will remove stale sweat whilst deodorants (which mask smells) and anti-perspirants (which reduce sweating) can help to prevent body odour.

Keep your hands and fingernails clean and well presented. Be sure to remove large rings and bracelets, which can easily become caught in the client's hair.

To do
■ Make a list of the most common infectious conditions that you could contract and pass on in the salon.   ■ Describe where you would go for medical advice for each of these conditions (e.g. to the doctor or to the pharmacist).   ■ Check the list with your supervisor and ask which ones should be reported.

A hairdresser's style of dress reflects attitudes to fashion and the design of the salon. Accessories such as jewellery, including earrings, brooches, hair ornaments and badges, must blend with the overall look.

Generally, clothes worn in the salon should be comfortably loose fitting, clean, neatly pressed and regularly mended. Cotton fabrics are often cooler to wear, but synthetics are generally more hard wearing.

If clients like the way that the hairdresser is dressed and like the hairdresser's own hairstyle, then they will have more confidence in their own finished hairstyle.

When hairdressers look presentable – neat, well groomed and clean – the client will have more confidence and is more likely to return and become a regular client.

Good posture is important too, because it looks better, as clothes will hang properly. It is also more healthy because the bones, muscles, tendons and ligaments will be held in their correct positions, avoiding undue stretching and strain.

To stand correctly

In order to stand correctly keep the feet hip-width apart, with the weight of the body equally on both legs and with the knees slightly bent. Hips and shoulders should be level and the head held up. Common faults are round shoulders, hollow back and weight held mostly on one foot so that shoulders and hips are tilted.

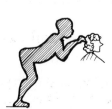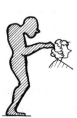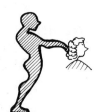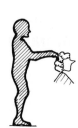

To sit correctly

In order to sit correctly the bones should form a right-angle at the hip and knee, with the hips and most of the thighs supported by the chair. Common faults are slouching (only the base of the spine in contact with the chair so that the back and thighs are not supported) and crossing the legs.

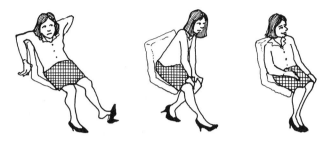

Regular exercise

All muscles need to be worked if they are to remain healthy. If unused, muscles will begin to weaken and waste away. Regular exercise, such as running, swimming, aerobics and brisk walking, will keep the muscles working correctly and help to maintain a good body shape. Exercise will also improve respiration, digestion and blood circulation, as well as relaxing nervous tension.

Test your knowledge

1 Why are cleanliness and good hygiene so important in the salon?
2 Name five infectious conditions that may be caught in the salon.
3 What should you do if you accidentally drop any of your tools on the floor?
4 List four points of salon hygiene that will minimise the danger of spreading infection.
5 What is the difference between disinfection and sterilisation?
6 What is the best way to clean and sterilise:
   ■ towels and gowns
   ■ combs and brushes
   ■ scissors?

Safety in the salon

Here is a brief list of the laws that affect you as an employee at work.

The Offices, Shops and Railway Premises Act (OSRPA) 1963

This Act says that your salon must be kept safe (against fire, electrical and chemical hazards) and clean and tidy (i.e. hygienic hazards). It means that you have to **obey the salon rules**.

The Employer's Liability (Compulsory Insurance) Act 1969

This requires employers to take out insurance on themselves and their employees for accidents to themselves and to clients.

Fire Precautions Act 1971

This is enforced by the local fire authority, usually the Fire Brigade. It states that all premises must have fire-fighting equipment in good working order, suitable for the type of fires likely to occur, and be readily available. It also states that the room contents should be arranged and doors left unlocked to enable a quick exit in the case of fire.

Health and Safety at Work Act 1974

This is enforced by Environmental Health Officers and Health and Safety Inspectors. It protects almost everyone involved in working situations. It states the responsibilities of the employer and the employees relating to:

- first-aid (emergency aid) arrangements and the reporting of accidents
- general health and safety
- enforcement of the Act.

Section 7 of this Act states

'It shall be the duty of every employee [you] at work –

- to take **reasonable care** for the health and safety of **himself or other persons** who may be **affected by his acts** or omissions at work.
- as regards any duty or requirement imposed on the employer or any other person by or under any of the relevant statutory provisions, to **co-operate with him** (the **employer**) so far as is necessary to enable that duty or requirements to be performed or complied with.'

The Reporting of Injuries, Diseases and Dangerous Occurrences Regulations 1985 (RIDDOR)

If you or your clients suffer from a personal injury at work then it must be reported in the salon's accident book. This is to inform your employer and so that serious injuries may be reported to the local Enforcement Officer.

The Control of Substances Hazardous to Health Act 1988 (COSHH)

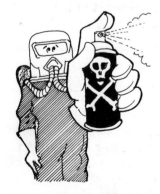

This is enforced by Health and Safety Inspectors. It is particularly relevant to the storage and use of hazardous chemicals such as hydrogen peroxide or perm lotions.

It applies not only to you but also to chemicals applied and sold to non-employees, i.e. **clients**.

The excellent leaflet *A Guide to Health and Safety in the Salon*, published by HMWA (The Hairdressing Manufacturers' and Wholesaler's Association Ltd) is available to all salons.

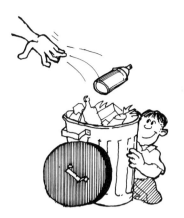

The Environmental Protection Act 1990

This Act States that hairdressing salon chemicals (i.e. 'waste') must be disposed of safely – i.e. **poured down the sink** (to dilute and remove them). **Never** put them in the dustbin where they could be found by children!

Electricity at Work Regulations 1990

This states that every electrical appliance in a work site must be tested at least every 12 months by a qualified electrician. A written record must be kept of these tests to be shown to the health and safety authorities upon inspection.

To do

- Find the address of your local Health and Safety Executive (HSE) office from the library and contact them to ask for up-to-date publications and information.

The Workplace (Health, Safety and Welfare) Regulations 1992

These have taken the place of most of the Offices, Shops and Railways Premises Act 1963, and require all at work to **maintain a safe and healthy working environment**. They apply very strongly to hairdressing salons.

The Manual Handling Operations Regulations 1992

These place upon all at work the duty to **minimise the risks from lifting and handling** objects.

The Personal Protective Equipment at Work Regulations 1992

These confirm the requirement for all employers to provide suitable and sufficient **protective clothing**, and for all employees to **use it when required**. This means wearing protective gloves and tinting aprons when colouring, bleaching, perming and straightening.

The Provision and Use of Work Equipment Regulations 1992

These impose upon the employer the duty to select equipment for use at work which is properly constructed, suitable for the purpose and kept in good repair. **Employers must also ensure that all who use the equipment have been adequately trained.** The requirement for competence to use salon tools and equipment is embodied within these hairdressing standards.

159

Salon hazards

Carelessness, tiredness or insufficient training can result in accidents such as those given in the table below.

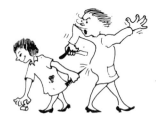

Accidents in the salon

Accident	Cause
Chemical burns	Spilt hydrogen peroxide Spilt permanent wave lotion or relaxers Use of incompatible chemicals (such as metallic dyes and hydrogen peroxide) on hair, creating enough heat to burn the skin
Physical burns	Electric tongs, hot brushes, hair dryers, accelerators or infra-red bulbs used near the skin
Scalds	Boiling water or steamers burning the skin
Allergies	Permanent dyes (used without a skin test), causing a reaction (contact dermatitis)
Cuts	Scissors, razors (see page 199 for disposing of detachable razor blades), broken glass
Infection	Little or no treatment of injuries Inadequate sterilisation of tools and equipment
Falls	Slippery floors caused by spillage of water, shampoo or grease, or obstructions left in the way such as boxes of stock or large shopping bags
Electric shock	Water and electricity coming into contact Electrical appliances poorly insulated
Poisoning	Drinking from incorrectly labelled bottles Inhaling dangerous vapours from chemicals such as ammonia
Fire	Incorrect handling of inflammable hairdressing chemicals such as ethyl acetate (nail polish remover) and hairspray Careless cigarette smoking

> **Remember**
>
> If you cannot rectify a hazard yourself, report it to your supervisor immediately.

Safety procedures

There are four main areas of salon safety of which you need to be aware.

1. Emergency procedures.
2. Using salon chemicals safety.
3. Controlling the salon environment.
4. Using electrical equipment safely.

Emergency procedures

You must know how to vacate your building quickly and safely in the case of fire, flood, gas leaks, suspicious packages or a bomb alert. You must be aware of where fire-fighting equipment is kept and know how to use it.

To do

Find your salon's:

- emergency exits
- nearest escape route
- nearest telephone (to ring the emergency services)
- fire-fighting appliances
- electricity mains switch
- gas mains tap
- water mains stopcock.

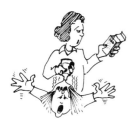

Using salon chemicals safely

Chemical substances are hazardous by:

- **inhalation** – breathing in fumes
- **ingestion** – swallowing them directly or by eating food while chemical is on the fingers
- **absorption** – through the skin or via the eyes
- **contact** – with the skin or eye surface (a chemical of this sort is known as an irritant).

Basic safety rules for storage of salon chemicals

- **Never use food or drink containers** to store any chemical product.
- Store products **at or below room temperature** in a dry atmosphere, never in direct sunlight.
- Keep products, particularly aerosols, **away from naked flames** or sources of heat.
- Take special care to **prevent children gaining access** to salon storage areas. Keep all products out of reach of children.

Mixing chemicals safely
- Follow the manufacturer's **instructions** exactly.
- **Dilute the product** according to the manufacturer's recommendations.
- **Never mix products** unless this is recommended by the manufacturer.
- Replace all caps and bottle tops immediately to **avoid spillage**. Make sure unused mixtures and empty containers are disposed of carefully.

Using chemicals safely
- Always wear **protective gloves** and protective **clothing** where indicated (see the chart below).
- Remember that prolonged and frequent use of non-hazardous products such as shampoos may cause dryness and sore skin. To avoid this wear protective gloves or use barrier cream and moisturiser as often as possible.
- Wipe and clean all surfaces where spillages occur.

Chemicals: hazards and precautions

Chemical	Health hazard	Precautions
All aerosols, including hairspray	Dangerous if inhaled excessively Flammable	Use in a well ventilated area Keep well away from lighted cigarettes Do not tamper with valves: the contents are under pressure and can explode in a fire
Setting lotions, mousses and gels	Potential irritant Flammable	Avoid eye contact Keep away from lighted cigarettes
Hydrogen peroxide	Irritant to skin and eyes	Always wear protective gloves Avoid contact with eyes and sensitive skin Replace cap immediately after use Do not allow to mix with other chemicals as it can react and become explosive
Bleaches	Dangerous if inhaled excessively Irritant to skin and eyes	Use in a well-ventilated area Wear protective gloves Avoid contact with eyes and sensitive skin
Perm lotions and relaxers	Irritant to skin and eyes	Wear protective gloves Avoid contact with eyes and sensitive skin
Perm neutralisers	Irritant to skin and eyes	Wear protective gloves Avoid contact with eyes and sensitive skin
Hair colours, tints and semi-permanents	Irritant to skin and eyes Can cause allergic reactions	Wear protective gloves Avoid contact with eyes and sensitive skin Always do a skin test before use

Controlling the salon environment

This means making sure that the salon does not become too hot or cold or full of dangerous fumes. The Health and Safety at Work Act 1974 states that the working temperature should be 16°C, 60.8°F, after the first hour. Precautions should also be taken to avoid salons becoming humid due to hair drying equipment and steam from hot water supplies, which can also make it difficult to work.

To do

Find out how to:

- operate the salon's heating system through the use of thermostats
- ventilate the salon by opening the windows or using the extractor fans.

The COSHH regulations also cover ventilation, especially when mixing chemicals (think about the smell when mixing powder bleach for instance), so make sure you mix products in a well **ventilated** area.

Remember that portable gas or paraffin heaters also need proper ventilation to prevent any build up of irritant gases.

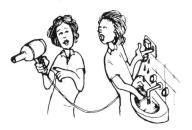

Using electrical equipment safely

The Electricity at Work Regulations 1990 state that electrical appliances must be tested regularly by a qualified person for safety, but it is also your responsibility to keep checking that all electrical equipment in the salon is in good condition.

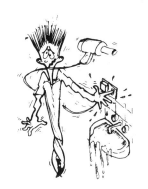

- Look at equipment to make sure that all the flexes and cables are not worn or faulty. Any flexes with worn insulation or any plugs that are broken or cracked should be replaced.
- Always make sure that electrical equipment is **stable** – check that hairdryers, tongs or hot brushes are safely stored on the work surface and not in places where they are likely to fall off.
- Never leave cables (dry flexes) where people could trip or **fall over** them.
- Check the **temperature controls** before using any equipment and make sure the filters at the back of the hairdryers are clear and free of dust or they will quickly overheat.
- Always switch off and disconnect equipment as soon as you have finished with it.

Electric shock

This occurs when a person's body completes an electrical circuit. The size of the shock depends on the size of the electrical current, and can vary from a slight tingling to a cardiac arrest (when the heart stops beating and breathing stops). It can happen:

- when a person touches bare wires on flexes or cables, or uses cracked plugs or switches
- through incorrect wiring or through a fault in the plug or appliance
- through touching a switch or plug with wet hands – water acts as a good conductor and electricity will flow through the person rather than through the circuit.

Remember		
E	= Earth	= green and yellow wire
N	= Neutral	= blue wire
L	= Live	= brown wire.

Wiring a plug

Make sure you know how to wire a plug correctly.

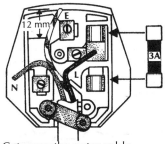

1 Cut away the outer cable, unscrew the cable grip and insert the cable

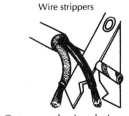

Wire strippers

2 Cut away the insulation using wire strippers

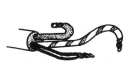

3 Twist the copper strands together

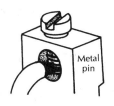

Metal pin

4 Insert each wire into the correct pin

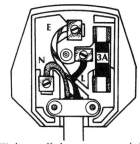

5 Tighten all the screws and the cable grip. Attach the plastic back

Test your knowledge

1 Who is responsible for enforcing government legislation regarding accident, emergency and evacuation procedures?

2 Which set of regulations particularly affects:
   - obeying the salon rules
   - salon insurance
   - fire extinguishers for use in the salon
   - emergency aid
   - the reporting of accidents
   - the storage and use of salon chemicals
   - disposing of salon waste chemicals safely
   - the safety and testing of electrical equipment
   - maintaining a safe salon
   - lifting and carrying heavy stock
   - wearing protective clothing at work
   - ensuring that salon equipment is safe and sound.

3 Where could you find out more information regarding these laws?

4 What are your responsibilities under COSHH?

5 Why is it important to keep the salon clean and tidy?

6 If the fire alarm sounded what should you do?

7 Name four ways in which salon chemicals can be harmful.

8 Why is it important to store chemicals at room temperature?

9 Why is it dangerous to allow children into the stock room?

10 Why should you always read the manufacturer's instructions before using salon products?

11 Name the chemicals used in the salon for which you always need to wear protective gloves.

12 Which salon products are known to cause allergies in some clients?

13 Which salon products or chemicals are known to be possible irritants to the eyes?

14 Some salon products are known to be more flammable than others. Name them.

15 Why is it important to be able to ventilate the salon properly?

16 Name all the different pieces of electrical equipment used in your salon and list which parts of them should be tested for safety.

17 What is an electric shock?

18 Give three reasons why electric shock can occur.

19 Why should you always be alert to salon hazards?

20 When should you ask your supervisor to deal with salon hazards?

21 Describe how to dispose of salon waste chemicals and why this is important.

22 Describe the types of records required and how they should be completed.

23 Why is a hairdresser's personal health and hygiene important in the salon?

24 Why is a hairdresser's personal appearance and conduct important to clients?

25 Describe how poor posture and deportment can be harmful to the hairdresser.

26 Name any infectious conditions that may need to be reported in the salon.

27 How should you avoid cross-infection from open cuts and abrasions?

Emergency aid

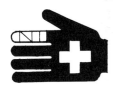

Emergency aid in the salon usually involves the treatment of minor accidental injuries. However, a qualified first-aider would be able to help with more serious injuries such as bone fractures or heart attacks before the patient is seen by a doctor. The aim of first aid is to prevent death or further damage to injured persons. If you have any doubt about an injury, always seek medical advice from a doctor or nurse at a health clinic or the casualty department at a hospital.

Common accidents and conditions in the salon

Accident/condition	Emergency aid action
Salon chemicals in the eye, e.g. perm lotions, bleaches, tints	Wash the eye with running water (under the tap if possible). Continue applying water to the eye until medical assistance is available
Salon chemicals on the skin, e.g. perm lotions, bleach	Flood the area with water to dilute and remove the chemical
Salon chemicals swallowed, e.g. chemicals placed in soft-drink containers and drunk by mistake	Drink 2–3 glasses of water. Seek medical advice immediately
Salon chemicals inhaled, e.g. strong bleach mixtures	Move the person to fresh air immediately. Seek medical advice if coughing, choking or breathlessness lasts longer than 10–15 minutes
Dry heat burns, e.g. from hairdryers, tongs, hot brushes, crimping irons	Hold affected area under running cold water or apply ice pack (5–10 minutes). Seek medical advice if necessary
Scalds, e.g. from hot water supplies or steamers	Hold affected area under running cold water or apply ice pack (5–10 minutes). Seek medical advice if necessary
Minor cuts	Apply pressure until bleeding stops. Avoid direct contact with blood because of the risk of infectious diseases such as AIDS and Hepatitis B. Wherever possible, ask clients to use a clean piece of cotton wool and apply pressure themselves, then throw the cotton wool into a plastic bag or bin afterwards.
Severe cuts	The blood flow from severe cuts should be stopped by applying pressure with either a clean towel or hands (covered with rubber gloves from the first-aid box). Phone for an ambulance immediately.
Electric shock	If someone is being electrocuted do not touch the person as you will be electrocuted yourself. Turn off the electricity immediately, either by turning off the switches or pulling out the plug. If breathing has stopped then artificial respiration will need to be applied by a qualified first-aid person. Phone for an ambulance straight away.
Client distress, e.g. fainting	This is caused by lack of oxygen to the brain. If someone feels faint put their head between their knees and loosen any tight clothing. If the person has fainted, raise the legs on a cushion so that they are higher than the head.

> **Remember**
>
> The RIDDOR Act states that all accidents must be reported in the accident register kept in the salon.

First-aid kits

All salons should provide a first-aid box (usually coloured green with a white cross) containing a first-aid kit. It should include:

- a first-aid guidance card
- individual assorted plasters (preferably waterproof)
- medium, large and extra large sterile dressings
- bandages (including a triangular bandage)
- sterile eye pads
- scissors
- tweezers
- safety pins
- antiseptic lotion

It is also advisable to keep disposable rubber or plastic gloves for dealing with wounds that are bleeding or weeping. Except in an emergency, aid should not be given without wearing these gloves because of the risk of AIDS and Hepatitis B.

To do

- Find out where the first aid kit is located in your salon.
- Check its contents and report to your supervisor if anything is missing.

More serious signs of distress, such as heart attacks, stopped breathing, epileptic fits or fractures (from falls) should be dealt with by a qualified first-aider. If you wish to qualify, contact your local St John's Ambulance who regularly run courses.

Test your knowledge

1 What is emergency aid?
2 When would a qualified first-aider be needed?
3 When would you need to seek medical advice or call an ambulance?
4 What items would you expect to find in a first aid box?
5 If perm lotion accidentally ran into your client's eye, what would you do?
6 How would you deal with a child who has accidentally swallowed some hydrogen peroxide?
7 If some bleach spills on to your client's neck, how would you remove it?
8 What is the best treatment for someone who is choking after inhaling a strong chemical?
9 What could cause a dry heat burn?
10 How should you treat a scald on the hand from boiling water?
11 If you accidentally cut your client's ear, how should the bleeding be stopped?
12 Why must you always wear gloves when treating a person with a severe cut?
13 What is the most important action to take if someone is being electrocuted?
14 Why is it important to raise a person's feet if they have fainted?

11 Setting and dressing short and long hair

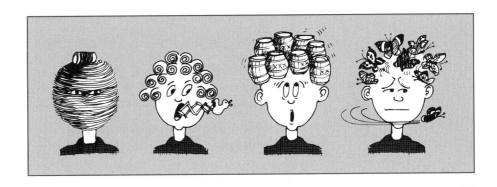

Setting hair can be just as exciting as blow-drying hair: the same set on short, medium or long hair can give you three completely different looks when you brush them through.

Deciding the style

Never say to the client 'What colour rollers [i.e. size] do you have?' You are the professional, and should be recommending not only what size of rollers but also what type of style will best suit the client. You would not go to the dentist and say which teeth you would like filled, would you?

Always consider the following points:

- **Is the set for any particular occasion?**
  Is the set for everyday wear or for a special event such as a party, dinner-dance or wedding?
- **How curly is the hair?**
  Curly hair (naturally curly or permed) may need to be straightened for a wavy look by using large rollers. Straight hair may need smaller rollers to produce a curl.
- **How long is the hair?**
  The longer the hair, the heavier it becomes, so if a client with long straight hair wants a curly look you will have to use smaller rollers.
- **How thick is the hair?**
  Clients with a lot of thick, textured hair will need larger rollers but those with a small amount of fine hair will need smaller rollers.

167

- **How bouncy is the hair?**
  'Bounciness' depends on the amount of elasticity in the hair, and clients with limp, lifeless hair (no elasticity) will need smaller rollers.

> **To do**
>
> ■ Re-read the section in Chapter 1 on designing a hairstyle to suit your client.
> ■ Make a short list of the rules that apply when setting (e.g. a client with a short neck will look better with an upswept, flicked style at the nape).

Hair growth patterns

The client's natural hair fall and movement can easily be seen when the hair is wet.

> **To do**
>
> ■ Re-read the section in Chapter 1 on hair growth patterns, then for your next client explain the difference between the natural hair fall (or parting) and the hair growth patterns (front hairline, crown area and nape areas) to your supervisor.

If you set the hair **with the natural fall** or hair growth pattern then the style will last longer and the client will find it easier to manage.

Why the shape of the hair can change through setting

> **Remember**
>
> Hair in its natural unstretched state is known as **alpha keratin**. Hair in its new, stretched (set) shape is known as **beta keratin**.

Setting, like blow drying, is a **temporary process** (unlike perming, which is a permanent process). This means that we can change the shape of the hair by making curly hair straight or straight hair curly – and if we do not like the result, we can quickly dampen down the hair and change it.

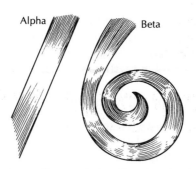

Naturally straight hair becomes curly, changing from alpha to beta keratin

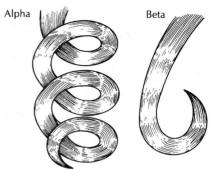

Naturally curly hair becomes straight, changing from alpha to beta keratin

> **To do**
>
> Re-read the section in Chapter 1 on hair structure. Make a note of which bonds in the cortex are broken during setting and blow drying, and the name of the protein in hair.

The temporary bonds in the cortex, which are broken during wet setting (also known as cohesive setting), allow the hair to be stretched even longer (up to half its length again).

Setting aids and products

Sets last much longer in dry atmospheres (like the Middle East) than in damp, humid atmospheres (like the United Kingdom), where they drop very quickly. This is because hair is **hygroscopic**, and the stretched beta keratin (the cohesive set) will gradually return to alpha keratin.

Setting aids such as setting lotion, sculpting lotions, moulding mists or gel coat the hair with a very fine film of plastic to stop moisture from being absorbed into the hair.

Setting aids are always applied to towel-dried hair; too much water in the hair would dilute the product.

Always check the manufacturer's instructions but, as a rule, most mousses and gels should be placed in the centre of the palm and then spread evenly over the hair with the fingers. Setting lotions must be sprinkled evenly all over the hair.

Some setting aids and products contain temporary colours (which wash out of the hair) such as silver, ash, coppers and reds. Use these only under supervision or once you have read Chapter 6. White hair will show the colours much more brightly than you expect.

To do

Find out which setting products in your salon are suitable for:

- fine hair
- coarse hair
- curly hair
- straight hair
- use on soft sets
- use on tight sets.

Hairsprays are used during combing out (or dressing) to control the hair and give more hold and body. They do this in the same way as setting aids, by coating the hair with a very fine film of plastic.

Static electricity

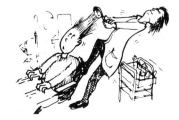

Hair dressings such as spray shines, waxes and creams are used on dry hair to help reduce static electricity, define the shape and finish off the style. They are only used a little at a time because the hair soon becomes over-greasy if too much is used.

Tools and equipment

Brushes

Brushes are used **before setting** to disentangle the hair before shampooing and during the client consultation, and **after setting** to remove all the roller marks and to dress the hair.

Flat brushes are normally used with open tufts or bristles which can go through the hair easily without tangling.

Combs

Combs are used to remove tangles (usually when the hair is wet), for parting and sectioning the hair and for combing out or dressing the hair.

Tail combs

These have a plastic or metal tail and usually one size of teeth. They are used for setting, when the tail is useful for tucking the ends of the hair cleanly round the roller.

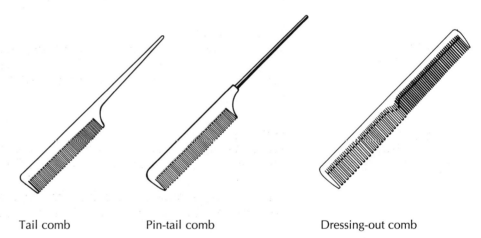

Tail comb   Pin-tail comb   Dressing-out comb

The larger teeth are used for disentangling the hair and for forming waves on finger waving, whereas the fine teeth are useful for back combing.

Rake combs

These combs are useful for disentangling hair after shampooing. They do not tear and stretch the hair because they have wide-spaced teeth.

Rollers

Setting rollers can be smooth or spiky. Spiky rollers hold the hair in place better, but can be difficult to keep clean and free from hairs. They can sometimes become tangled in the hair if they are not taken out carefully, and can cause dents or ridges on porous hair.

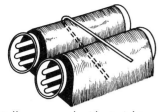

Rollers secured with straight pin

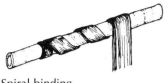

Spiral binding

Most rollers are held in place with either **straight** pins or **setting** pins.

Different-sized rollers are available for various effects, and they are often colour coded. Generally, the smaller the roller, the tighter the curl.

Molten Brown curlers are long, foam-filled curlers that can be used to achieve corkscrew, spiral curls.

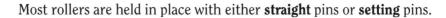

To do

- Look at all the sizes of setting rollers in your salon and make a note of the colour code for each size. The smaller the curler the tighter the curl produced.

Pins and clips

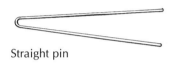

Straight pin

Straight pins
Straight, strong pins are made of metal and must never be used during perming, as they will react with the perm lotion and discolour the hair.

They are used to secure rollers **during setting** and for **dressing long** hair.

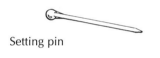

Setting pin

Plastic setting pins
These can also be used to hold rollers in place during setting, but they do tend to distort the hair and leave marks.

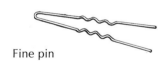

Fine pin

Fine hairpins
These are mainly used during **combing out**, especially when putting up long hair. They are often available in several shades to match the client's hair colour. They are not very strong and will hold only small amounts of hair.

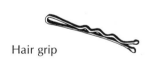

Hair grip

Hairgrips
Hairgrips, like fine hairpins, are available in a variety of colours to match the client's hair colour, and are mostly used for **long hair** dressings.

The flat prong is always placed flat to the head, and the ends of both prongs are covered with plastic to prevent them from scratching the client's scalp.

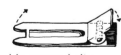

Double-pronged clip

Double-pronged clips
These can be made of metal or plastic and are usually used for **securing pin curls**.

Hair nets

Nylon setting nets are usually triangular in shape and are used to keep **rollers and pin curls in place** while the client is under the dryer. Ear shields may also be used to protect the client's ears under the hairdryer, but they must be clean and sterile.

Hood dryers

These are used to dry the hair where rollers or pin curls have been used, or for natural drying under a slow speed setting. They may be part of a drying bank, attached to the wall, or portable (free-standing) and moved to the dressing position. Always remember to show your client how to use the dryer controls.

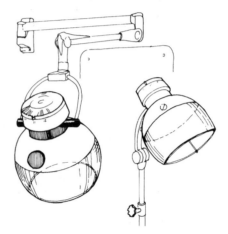

Using mirrors when setting

During setting you will need to use your mirror to check that the sections and partings are in the right place. You also need your mirror to check the shape of the hairstyle for balance, and to make sure there are no breaks or holes in the finished work.

Setting techniques (cohesive setting)

Once the hair has been shampooed, towel dried and any setting aids applied, then the hair must be combed to find the natural fall.

Decide the style with your client. Then choose the size of rollers and decide whether you need to use any pin curls.

The final set is call the '**pli**' (pronounced 'plee').

To do

■ Look up Chapter 1 to find out how to gown and protect your client for setting, including any changes needed for using temporary colours.

Sectioning

Sectioning allows you to work methodically (step-by-step), and without being muddled.

The size and areas of section will depend on what you are doing. For example, **pin curls** need **small square sections** but **rollers** need **larger oblong sections**.

Remember

Sections for rollers must have clean lines and be **just a little smaller** than the roller size.

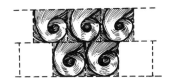

Sections for pin curls

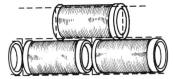

Sections for rollers

To section the hair, comb the hair flat then use your tail comb to **draw a clean line** with the end of the teeth of the comb along the scalp. The hair should then be parted in two. Hold the hair apart with one hand then comb the hair down either side to **create a clean parting**.

If you are rollering, place the roller on the hair to measure the width of the section (it should be just shorter than the roller) and **make a second parting** parallel to the first. To complete the oblong section use the **tail** end of the comb (without teeth) underneath the roller to complete the third line of the section.

To do
■ Practise making clean, neat sections for rollers. Sections must be good for setting, but perfect for perming (the sections for perming are the same but smaller).

Setting with rollers

Rollers are used to create volume and lift in the finished style.

It is easier to start at the top of the head, but always plan your pli in your mind before starting. Think about which **size of rollers** will be used on **which area** of the head and **where** the pin curls will be placed.

Once the section has been taken, comb the hair smoothly and evenly, without using any undue tension or pulling too much. Take the roller and wind the hair evenly and cleanly down to the scalp so that the roller sits on its base, then secure it with a pin.

Remember

The roller size chosen for each pli (set) will vary according to:

■ the style chosen
■ the amount of curl already in the hair
■ the length and amount of hair
■ the elasticity of the hair (some hair has very little elasticity and needs smaller rollers than usual).

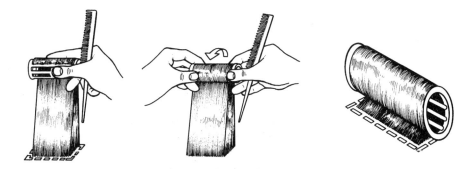

Never allow the metal pins to touch the client's scalp or face as they become hot under the dryer and can burn.

Rollers can also be placed off their base if a softer, flatter effect is required.

Remember

Rollers placed **on their base** give **root lift**. Rollers placed **off** their base give **no root lift**.

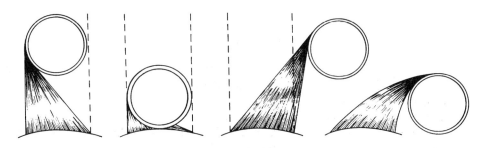

173

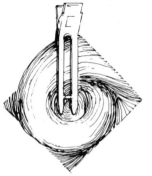

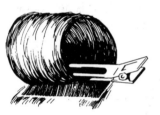

The most common type of pin curl: a barrelspring curl

Stand-up barrel curl

Setting with pin curls

Pin curls are used to produce **height**, **wave movement** and **curl** in the finished dressing. They are usually secured with double-pronged clips, but care must be taken when securing them so that they do not become distorted.

Pin curls are made by turning around the ends of small, square sections of hair using the fingers to form a curl.

When you are working at the back and sides of the head, always ask your client to move their head forwards or to the side when necessary so that you can work properly.

Stand-up barrel curls
These are formed to give the same effect as you would achieve from using a roller, often where the space between the rollers is too small for another roller to fit.

Flat barrelspring curls
These pin curls are placed flat to the head to produce **soft curls**.

If one row of pin curls is placed in one direction and the next row is placed in the opposite direction, it is called **reverse pin curling**. These curls will brush out to form a wave movement.

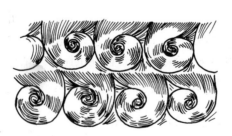
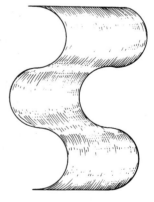

Reverse pin curls

Clockspring curls
These are small, flat pin curls with a closed centre. The ends of the curl form a small closed circle with each loop becoming larger. They are normally used in the nape to produce **tight curls**.

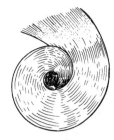

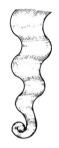

Clockspring curl

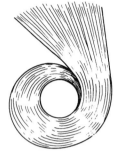

Long-stemmed pin curl

Long-stemmed pin curls

These are useful for creating **soft curl** results **around the hairline**. As only the ends of the hair are curled they are often secured to the skin with special sticky tape.

Finger waving

Finger waving is a way of moulding the hair with your fingers and salon comb to form a series of 'S'-shaped movements in the hair. It is best done on wet hair, but is also used on dry hair during combing out.

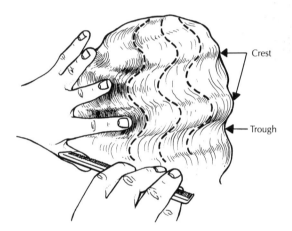

Points to remember for finger waving

Finger waving is best done on medium length, tapered hair that is **not too curly**.

- Keep the hair **very wet**. Use a thick setting gel to help form the waves.
- Always find the client's **natural fall** or parting and any natural wave movement, and finger wave **with** this movement. The hair should just fall into place.
- Use the **wide teeth** of the salon comb to comb the hair as these teeth penetrate the hair better.
- To form the 'S'-shaped movements start by combing the hair into a semi-circular shape, to form the **trough** of the wave. Then hold the hair in the centre of the wave in place with the middle and index fingers, while you comb the next section of hair into a semi-circular shape (in the opposite direction) to form the **crest** of the wave.

To do
■ Practise finger waving on any clients who can spare the time before setting their hair.

Variations of sets

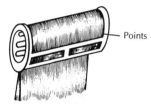

Croquinole winding

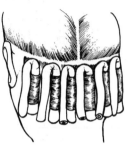

Spiral wind: in position

There are many different ways of placing both rollers and pin curls to create different effects.

In normal setting the hair is wound from points (ends) to roots. This is called **croquinole winding**.

If you have long hair and wish to achieve a tight curl at the roots as well as the ends, then you can use Molten Browners and spirally wind the hair. For best results, use end papers on towel-dried hair and secure the root end by bending the curler over.

To do
■ Practise spiral winding on long hair.

Dry Setting

Remember

- ■ Dry sets work by turning the moisture in the hair into steam so always allow the hair to **cool thoroughly before dressing out.**
- ■ **Fine hair** and **curly hair** take a **stronger curl** than thick straight hair.
- ■ **One-length straight hair drops the curl** quickly because of its weight.
- ■ **Larger sections** are taken when dry setting to achieve a more **casual look.**

Fashion setting may be achieved on **wet**, **damp** or **dry hair**. The wetter the hair, the firmer and more long-lasting the set. Hair that is very wet and long takes a long time to dry, so more casual looks are achieved on clean dry hair. A **thermal (heat active) styling lotion** is then evenly applied and the hair may be set with either:

- **velcro rollers** (which do not need pins), re-sprayed with lotion, and placed under a hairdryer (for 10–15 minutes) or
- **heated rollers**, which cool down after 10–15 minutes.

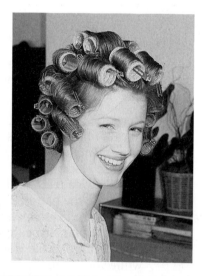

Setting tight curly hair

Naturally tight curly hair is normally set after either temporary straightening (soft or hard pressing) or permanent straightening (relaxing) to create a modern fashion look. Hair that has been permed to create a tight curly look may also be set when it is wet to create a softer style.

Here are some examples of different pli patterns. Notice that all the rollers are placed into a brickwork pattern – rollering in lines will only produce gaps and breaks in the comb out.

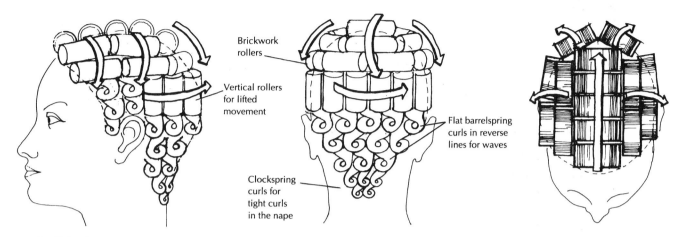

Brickwork rollers

Vertical rollers for lifted movement

Flat barrelspring curls in reverse lines for waves

Clockspring curls for tight curls in the nape

Back off the face

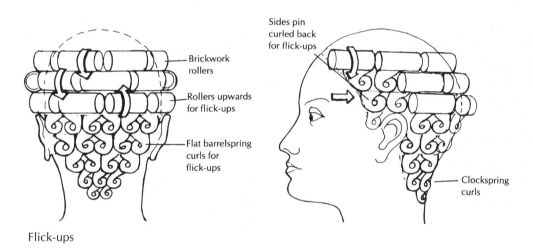

Brickwork rollers

Rollers upwards for flick-ups

Flat barrelspring curls for flick-ups

Flick-ups

Sides pin curled back for flick-ups

Clockspring curls

Remember

The **more rollers** you use, the greater the amount of **curl and wave movement** you will achieve and the longer the set will last.

Always use **even tension** on the rollers or they will become lop-sided and the hair will fall off the sides.

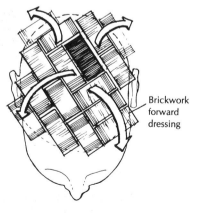

Brickwork forward dressing

Forward onto the face

Combing out (dressing the hair)

Check that the hair is dry, then allow the hair to cool for a few minutes before removing the rollers. Always take the rollers out from the **underneath first** if the hair is long or it may become tangled.

Some clients prefer a perfectly finished dressing, others like a more casual result. The final dressing is what the client is paying for, so **make sure that they are satisfied** with the result.

You must first brush the hair in **all directions** to remove any roller marks, then brush in the **direction of the style**. Only back comb or back brush where necessary.

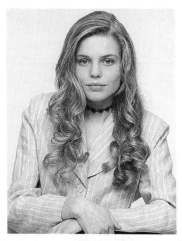

To do

Re-read the section in Chapter 3 on finishing products. Hair sprays, gels, waxes, pomades, dressing creams, moisturisers, serums and activators may also be used before and after dressing out hair. Check all your manufacturer's instructions regarding the use of finishing products – many have to be used sparingly.

Back brushing and back combing

Both of these techniques work by pushing the cuticle scales apart so they tangle with each other. Both methods give lift and volume to the hairstyle.

Hold the points or ends of the hair firmly in one hand and either back comb underneath or back brush on top. Then gently smooth over the top to give a neat finish.

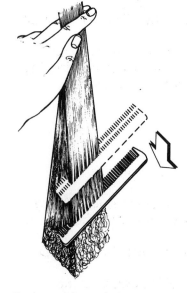

Back-combing technique

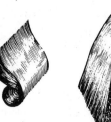

Existing curl

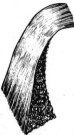

Create lift

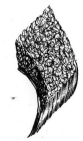

Back brush top of mesh

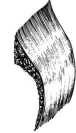

Smooth over with comb

Always stand some distance away from your client to check the finished result, especially the shape. Look for any breaks or gaps in the dressing and smooth over if necessary.

Check the overall shape, looking at the back, sides and front. Does it frame the face properly? Remember that the client sees only the front area. It is the most important part of the dressing.

Hairspray and aerosol spray shines may now be used to finish the work and hold the shape.

To do

■ Practise showing clients the back of their hair using the back mirror. It should be held so that you can **both** see the back view.

Dressing out long hair

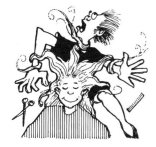

Many hairdressers worry about working with long hair but with planning and practice it will become easy.

To do

■ Using your style book and a long-haired practice head, follow the instructions in this book and practise plaiting, a pleat and a roll. Ask your supervisor to comment on your work.

Client consultation

- Use your **style book** to discuss the style with your client and select the type of dressing most suitable.
- Discuss the **occasion** with your client – is it for evening wear, or for a wedding (will you need extra holding sprays for bad weather?)
- Discuss the **clothes** your client will be wearing. Do they have a high or a low neckline? Will the hairstyle balance with the clothes?
- How much **time** will you need to dress the style, the client will not want to be late for a special occasion.
- Discuss the **cost**. Many salons charge extra for putting long hair up.
- For a very special occasion such as a wedding, have a **rehearsal** dressing beforehand to make sure you know exactly what the client wants.

General points

You will need to consider the following:

- **The shape of the head** – e.g. if it is flat at the back more hair will be needed there to balance it.
- **The shape of the face** – e.g. if a round or square face is exposed by the hair being dressed up then a few tendrils of hair around the face may be used to soften it.
- **The amount of hair** – does the client have enough hair for the dressing or will a hairpiece be needed?
- **Hair growth patterns** – e.g. a widow's peak could be exposed if the client's hair is pulled back, it may be softer to take the hair to the side.

- **Hair texture** – fine frizzy hair may need wax, moisturisers or dressing cream to smooth it. Strong coarse hair may need a strong styling lotion for control.
- **Hair structure** – e.g. if the hair is very straight will it need to be set first? If the hair is very curly will it need to be straightened first?

Preparation

Gowning up

Remove any large earrings or necklaces that the client is wearing, in case they become entangled in the client's long hair.

Freshly washed hair is difficult to dress so use a **styling lotion** during drying for control.

During dressing, products such as dressing creams (to remove frizz) wax and gels (to define the shape) and finishing spray (to hold the hair) are invaluable – but use them **sparingly**.

Equipment

Covered elastics, and grips with **covered ends** are used to prevent hair damage, and should be kept to a minimum. This is because they should not show in the finished dressing and too many grips would be too heavy to wear comfortably.

Ornamentation

If you are using ornaments, such as combs, slides, flowers, ribbons or head-dresses, in your dressing choose them carefully and make sure they balance the style rather than overwhelm it

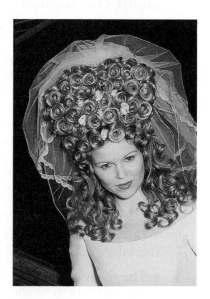

Dressing hair down

To dress out **straight hair**, simply brush it in place using your hands to create a smooth finish.

To dress out **curly hair** – use your fingers or an afro comb to shape the hair. If you use a brush it will become frizzy.

Dressing hair up

Plaiting – The hair is normally blow dried first using a styling product for control. Never over-dry the hair – it will lose its natural moisture content

If the hair is to be twisted or plaited, it must be brushed or combed smoothly and then divided into equal amounts. Secure the hair with special elasticated bands.

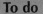
To do

Use the illustrations below to practise making twists and plaits.

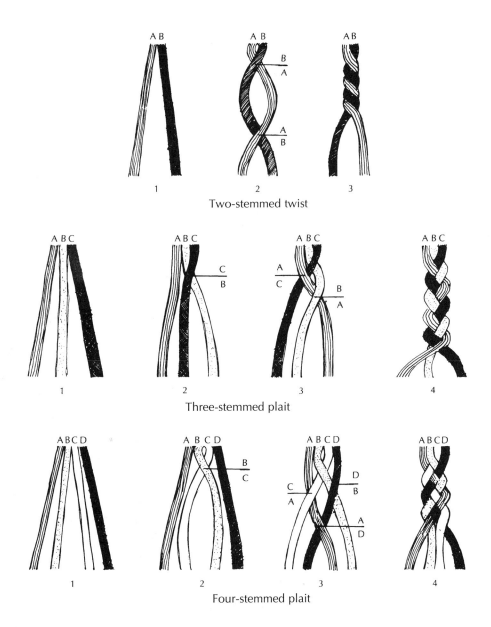

Two-stemmed twist

Three-stemmed plait

Four-stemmed plait

French plait

A French plait is a three-stemmed plait, best done on dry hair. Starting at the front hairline, take a small triangular section and split the hair into three equal sections.

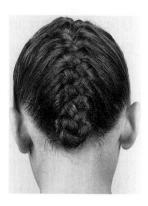

Work up to Diagram 3 of the three-stemmed plait diagram, then take another small section of hair from the **right-hand** hairline and add it to B/A. Pull the plait tight to the scalp. Next, take another small section from the **left-hand** hairline, keeping the hair combed smooth to the head, and add it to C/B. Pull the hair tight to the scalp. Continue adding small sections of hair to the plait until the French plait is completed.

Pleats and rolls

Wet, dry, or damp set the hair first on medium or large rollers to give some lift. The wetter the hair the more curly it will be.

A pleat

A pleat is a **vertical** roll of hair worn at the back of the hair.

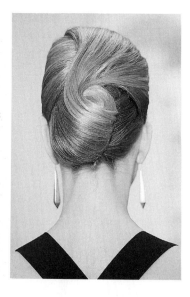

Method
- Back-comb or back-brush to create volume, control and hold the hair together. Back-comb **underneath** the hair section at the roots and a little the mid length and ends (Figure 1).
- Leave out the top section and brush or comb (using the wide teeth) one side of the hair smoothly towards the centre back. Secure with a line of **interlocking** grips, placing one grip over the end of the last, firmly to the scalp. Finish the line of grips just under the crown area. If you are right handed, it is easier to secure the left side first (Figure 2).

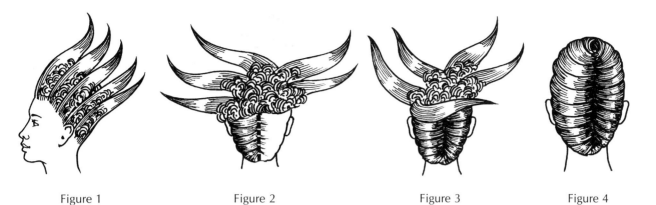

Figure 1   Figure 2   Figure 3   Figure 4

- Brush or comb the other side of the hair across towards the centre back. Check that the pleat is in the middle, then twist or fold this hair under and secure firmly with grips or pins, making sure that they do not show (Figure 3).
- Smooth over the top hair and blend it in with the pleated back hair completing the pleat smoothly and tucking the ends in (Figure 4). Grip it firmly, then check the front of the dressing for balance and shape. If the hair needs lifting use a pin or the end of a tail comb carefully so as not to disturb the hair that is already secured. Use any finishing spray as desired. Check that no pins or grips are visible.

A roll

A roll is a **horizontal** roll of hair, which may be worn at the back, sides or top of the hair.

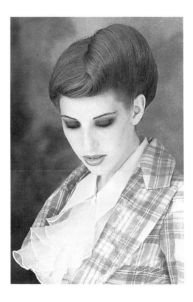

Method
- Back-comb or back-brush to create volume, control and hold the hair together. Back-comb **underneath** the hair section of the finish direction of the roll, both at the roots and a little at the mid-lengths and ends (Figure 1).
- Smooth over the top hair in the direction of the finished dressing and then decide on the height of the finished roll. Place a row of **interlocking** hair grips, placing one grip of the end of the last, firmly to the scalp in a line just under where the roll will be placed (Figure 2).

183

- Starting at one side of the head, brush or comb the hair up towards the grips and fold the hair over. Tuck it under to form a horizontal roll and grip it firmly as you work from one side to the other. Work around the head, checking in the mirror for shape and balance before you complete the result. Check that no pins or grips are visible (Figures 3 and 4).

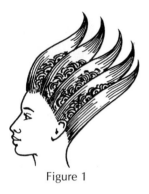

Figure 1

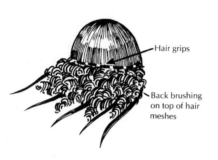

Hair grips

Back brushing on top of hair meshes

Figure 2

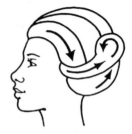

Figure 3

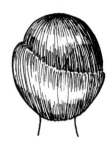

Figure 4

Setting faults and corrections

Fault	Cause	Correction
'Fish hooks' or buckled, frizzy ends	Ends of hair not wound smoothly around the rollers	Try using electric tongs to smooth out the hair. 'Fish hooks' will disappear as soon as the hair is wetted down
Hair not dry	Incorrect checking	Replace rollers and re-dry the hair under the dryer. If brushed through, then dry with a hand dryer and small circular brush
Hair not curly enough	Rollers too large	Use electric tongs to tighten the curl
Hair too curly	Rollers too small	Use hand dryer and brush to stretch the hair straighter
Hair is greasy and lank	Conditioner left in the hair or too much spray shine applied	The hair must be re-shampooed and set again
Hair is flyaway and full of static electricity	Too much shampoo used, or the hair is naturally flyaway	Apply a little spray shine to the hair. Use a setting aid next time
Holes and breaks in the hair in final comb out	Too few rollers. Not enough brushing or combing out	Re-back comb or back brush the area of hair

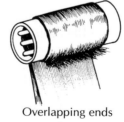

Overlapping ends

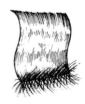

'Fish hooks'

Test your knowledge

1 What effect does the size of rollers have on the finished style?
2 What are the benefits of using too many rather than too few rollers when setting?
3 What are the effects of using
   - small rollers
   - large rollers
   - small rollers and clockspring pin curls
   - large rollers on top and smaller rollers underneath?
4 Why is the natural fall and root movement so important when designing the pli?
5 What happens to the temporary bonds in the cortex during cohesive (wet) setting?
6 Why does a set collapse on a damp, misty day?
7 List and compare different types of styling and drying equipment for use on tight curly, wavy and straight hair.
8 Describe which of the following products:
   - setting lotion
   - sculpting or moulding mists or lotions
   - mousse
   - gel

   would be suitable for setting fine hair/coarse hair/tight curly hair/wavy hair/straight hair/soft sets/tight sets.
9 Why should set hair sections be brushed out thoroughly before dressing and styling the hair?
10 List and compare different types of equipment and finishing products for use on tight curly, wavy and straight hair to achieve various looks.
11 Describe the type of products, equipment and ornamentation used for dressing tight curly, wavy, and straight long hair into different styles.

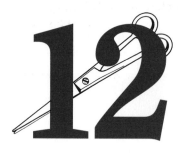

12 Modern men's barbering techniques

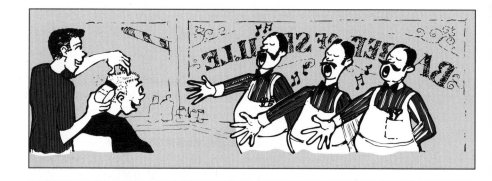

Men's barbering includes being able to cut **different short layered looks** (including various neckline shapes) and being able to cut beards, moustaches and sideburns into shape.

To do

■ Read Chapter 4, and test your knowledge before reading this chapter.

Short layered looks

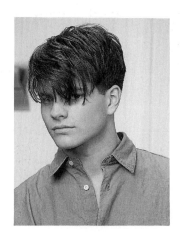

Technically, a man's haircut does not need to match perfectly in the way that a woman's haircut does. It is judged visually, i.e. the finished outline shape must look perfect

Head analysis

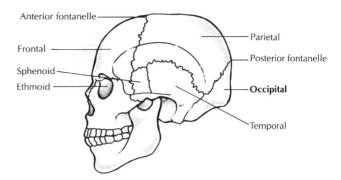

The bones of the head

Head shapes

A **man's occipital bone** tends to be **flatter** than a woman's occipital bone. Therefore, when you are cutting take the **weight** line **below the occipital bone** to make sure that the hair doesn't stick out

Face shapes

Square faces do not suit hard, sharp lines – use a finer graduation around the edges of the haircut for softness.

Round, softer, faces can take hard, sharp lines around the edges.

Hair growth patterns

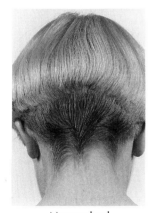

Nape whorl

Double crown – never cut hair too **short** on a double crown: it will stick up on end!

Neckline shapes – a **nape whorl** may be **tapered** into the back neckline, i.e. with **no line** cut around the bottom neckline

Back hairlines

Normal hairlines that grow down may be cut either **square or round** by using the scissors or the clippers **turned over**, depending on the clients' requirements. Generally, an uneven hairline is best left longer so that the hair can be cut evenly around it.

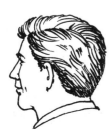

Round neckline

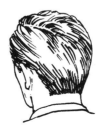

Square neckline

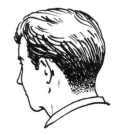

Tapered neckline

Front hairlines

Cowlicks are better left longer and styled the way the hair grows.

Male pattern baldness or receding hairlines generally suit a shorter haircut, rather than having a long piece of hair trailing over the top – but use **good communication** skills here before cutting it off – the client may like it.

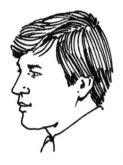 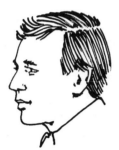 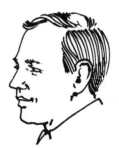 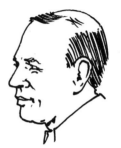 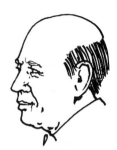

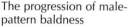

The progression of male-pattern baldness

Cicatrical alopecia or scarring, where the hair does not grow, should not be exposed – leave the hair longer to cover over.

Limitations

Remember

Always check for the presence of added hairpieces, such as a toupée, **before** you start cutting.

Hair structure

Straight fine hair must be cut carefully during scissors over comb work especially, or 'steps' will appear. Always **keep the comb and scissors moving** up and out (away from the head). If you have to remove a step, try chipping or pointing into it with the tips of your scissors to remove the line.

Wavy or tight curly hair is best club cut to reduce the curl. Short, afro hair is best cut out freehand with scissors or clippers (without a guard which could become entangled in the hair).

To do

■ Read the table on cutting tools and techniques in Chapter 4. Ask your supervisor to test you orally on which tools are used on wet and which on dry hair.

Hair texture

Coarse hair may need to be thinned, razored, tapered or texturised to **decrease** its weight and to achieve the correct shape.

Fine hair needs to be club or blunt cut to **increase** its weight and make it appear thicker.

Body build

If the client is very **tall**, don't crop the hair too short or cut a 'flat-top'. Leave some weight in the hair to balance the body.

Cutting tools

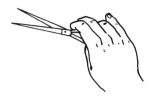

Correct way to hold scissors for regular cutting

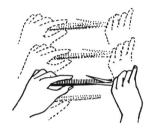

Turning the comb upward

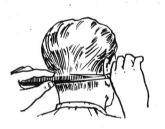

Using scissors and comb

Scissors

Most hairdressers use $4\frac{1}{2}$ to 5-inch **scissors** for cutting women's hair, and use only half an inch of the blade for cutting. Men's haircuts often take about 20 minutes, and therefore you need **longer blades** ($5\frac{1}{2}$ to 6 inches) to cut **more quickly**.

Thinning scissors are used for blending in weight lines and for softening hard lines, by being inserted at the ends of the hair.

To do
■ Practise holding your scissors and opening and closing the top blade with the back of your hand towards you. This is the only way you can cut the hair short enough during barbering.

Combs

Cutting combs are normally used for most cutting hair but **thin flexible barber's combs** are needed to cut around the ears and necklines for really short cuts.

Clippers

Electric clippers are used extensively for men's barbering techniques and so need to be kept **clean** and **well maintained**. The clipper blades need to be oiled or sprayed with clipper oil (this is an antiseptic oil) between clients, and must be kept free of cut hairs. If clippers pull hair, try cleaning and adjusting them.

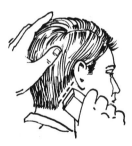

Outlining right side of neck

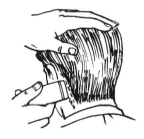

Outlining left side of neck

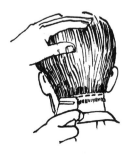

To produce a square nape line, turn clipper over on its cutting edge

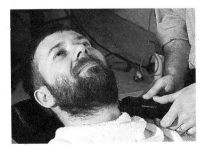

Outlining a beard

Remember
Health and safety   The **bottom**, static, **blade** of the clippers should always be **further forward** than the top, moving, blade. If the top blade comes too far forwards you could cut someone's skin, so be extra careful when clippers are turned over for lining out. Always put on the blade guard when clippers are not in use.

Remember

Health and safety
Always **change your razor's disposable blade** in front of the client so that your hygiene practises can be observed

Safety razors

Open razors with **disposable blades** are used for **hairline shaping** (lining out) and **removing unwanted hair outside the desired outline shape**. The best way to do this is to use a piece of cotton wool with warm water and shampoo to soften the hairs first, then stretch the skin tight before removing the hairs with the razor.

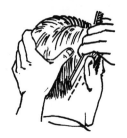

Shave outline below ear

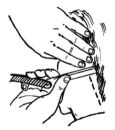

Shave left side of neck using backhand stroke

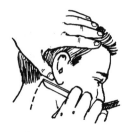

Clean neck below ear

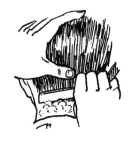

To achieve a square or round hairstyle, shaving or precision outlining is required

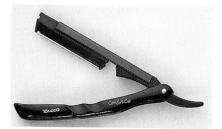

To do

■ Ask your supervisor for the salon's policy on how your used disposable razor blades (sharps) are disposed. Remember they are very dangerous pieces of equipment.

Nozzles

Nozzle attachments for hairdryers are always used for drying men's hair because they concentrate and direct the air flow onto the small section of short hair.

Neck brushes

These are used **continually during cutting** men's hair, not just at the end of the haircut, to constantly remove the tiny pieces of cut hair which would otherwise stick to the face or neck.

Preparation of client

Gowning up

Gowning up correctly is as important for male clients as it is for women. **Cutting collars** are particularly useful, especially when a strip of cotton wool is inserted between them and the client's neckline, to prevent hairs from falling down the client's neck.

Positioning yourself

Make sure that you are the correct height for the client. If a hydraulic chair is used pump it up or lower it to the correct working position before you start. If you are too tall for the client and you have to bend down – bend from the knees, keeping your back straight and working at a 90° angle to the client.

Positioning your client

Make sure that the client is **sitting level** (without his legs crossed) and that you are **working to his natural head position** (he must not be reading a book).

Preparing the hair

It is always better to work on clean, wet, freshly shampooed hair so that you can **see the natural fall clearly** and that all hair products have been removed. If the client does not want his hair washed and wet cutting techniques such as razor cutting are required, then spray the hair with warm water from a water spray.

Confirming the style

Once you have considered all the **critical influencing factors** (head and face shape, hair growth pattern and hair limitations) then you must confirm both the style and the length of the style with the client.

Cutting short layered looks

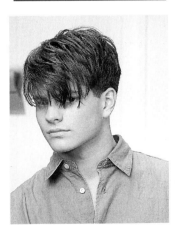

Scissor over comb and clipper over comb

Method
Sub-divide the head so that you can work on one area at a time. It is easiest to do the back first, then each side, and lastly the top and front.

The back
- **Start with your weight line**, cutting it horizontally to the required length. You may then work either down from the weight line to the neckline or from the neckline up to the weight line.
- **Removing a little hair at a time**, always **keep your** scissor over comb or clipper over comb **work moving**.
- The angle of your comb (which is always underneath your scissors or clippers) must be at the same angle as the head and parallel to it. The comb is always **moved up and out** away from the head so that the hair will join up with the weight line.
- **Start with a larger comb** to cut your weight line and change to your **finer barber's comb** for the short **underneath hair**.

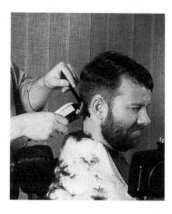 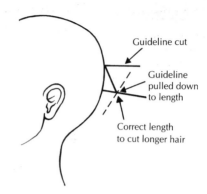

Taking guideline to length

- Always **take your cut guide line to your new length of hair** to be cut (not the other way around). This is sometimes called a travelling guide.
- You can **alter the closeness** of a clipper cut by **adjusting the blades** (normally by flicking a small switch on the side) to vary between 1/20 mm for the closest to 3 mm for the longest.
- **Clipper guards** may also be used to vary the length of the cut. The sizes are:

$$\begin{array}{lll} 1 & \text{or} & \frac{1}{16}'' \text{ (the shortest)} \\ 2 & \text{or} & \frac{1}{8}'' \\ 3 & \text{or} & \frac{1}{4}'' \\ 4 & \text{or} & \frac{3}{8}'' \text{ (longer hair)} \\ & & \frac{1}{2}'' \\ & & 1'' \end{array}$$

depending on the manufacturer.
- When you are cutting very short necklines **clipper across the head to cross-check the cut** as hair grows in all directions. If the hair grows upwards you will need to **clipper the hair down in the opposite direction**.
- An **undercut** style is where the hair is **clippered off underneath** and either layered or all one length on top. Section off the longer hair first, then clipper off the underneath hair before cutting the top hair to shape.

Other layering techniques

Layering techniques may also be adopted for styles

- with a parting
- with a fringe
- where the ears are exposed, or when the ears are covered
- to include natural hair growth patterns such as a double crown or cowlick.

Styles without a parting

These may be worn

- back off the face
- forwards onto the face
- brushed across to either side.

Remember

Always **protect the ears** by covering with either your comb or your hand during cutting.

The cutting is always the same on top – i.e. it is held at 90° and perfectly even when checked in every direction.

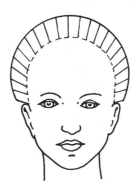
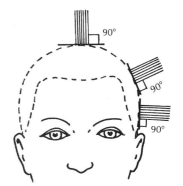

Hair cut without a parting

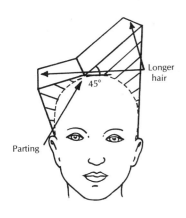

Hair cut with a parting

Styles with a parting

These normally have **longer hair on either side of the parting** to weigh the hair down. The hair is over-directed and held at 45°, not 90°, to create the length. The longer length weight line is created first and then the shorter layers are held at 45° and blended in to match.

Styles without a fringe

In these styles the hair is worn either back off the face or over to the side.

Styles with a fringe

These are when the hair is styled forward onto the face. To cut the hair with or without a fringe the front hair may be the same length as the top or a little longer, but still matching the layers.

The longer front hair is needed for blow drying back into a 'quiff' or 50s style, or if the fringe needs to cover a high forehead. Always texturise or 'chip into' (chipping is the same as pointing) the ends of a fringe to create softness on a man's haircut.

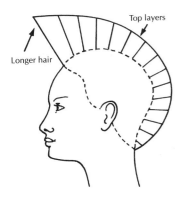

Hair left longer at front for a fringe or quiff

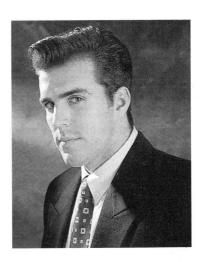

Styles with ears exposed

In such styles the hair is cut around the ear against the natural hairline. Always look at the **distance between this hairline and the ears** – there should **not be a large gap or space**. If the natural hairline is higher than the ears leave the hair a little longer to reduce the gap. Check the length of the sides with your client – does he want sideburns, a straight line or a pointed shape?

Side shapes

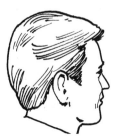
Pointed shape

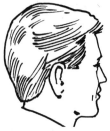
Straight shape

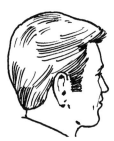
Sideburns

Once you have created the shape you may have to remove any unwanted hair with an open razor.

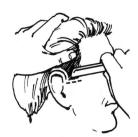
Shaving right sideburn to proper length

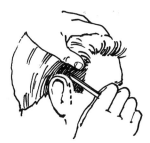
Shave over ear

Styles where the ears are covered

These also need careful cutting. **Never pull the hair tight or use tension** over the ears because the hair will lift up and become shorter when you let go! Just comb the hair evenly and cut it freehand to achieve the correct length.

Completing the cut

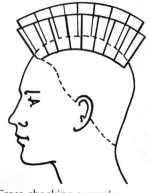
Cross checking a man's haircut

Cross checking a man's haircut

The difference between checking a man's haircut and a woman's haircut is that you should only cross-check a man's cut **vertically**. You do not cut the **corners off** as you would for a woman's cut. **The result should be more square than round.**

To **check the shape and balance** look at the man's **profile** from all angles, not just through the mirror. Place a **white towel over your shoulder** (unless the hair is white, when you should use a dark towel) to give a clear background and to see the shape properly.

Finishing off

Always ask the client if he is satisfied with the result and show him the back with the back mirror.

Although you have continually used the neck brush throughout the service, finally **check that he is free from all excess hair cuttings** once you have finished.

Styling products – if you are drying off the hair and need more control use an even distribution of a light blow-dry spray.

To do

■ Show the client how much product to use on his hair. Many clients use too much and often suffer from flaking scalps.

Once the hair is dry you can give a final shine or polish by using

● dressing cream (which is lighter than wax) for fine light-coloured hair
● wax for darker, heavier hair.

For illustrations of traditional and alternative haircuts for men, see the colour photographs between pages 196 and 197.

Test your knowledge

1 Describe the differences between cutting techniques and layering techniques and how they can be used to achieve a variety of layered looks.
2 List the cutting techniques that should be used on wet hair and the ones that should be used on dry hair.

Cutting beards, moustaches and sideburns

Fashions and trends in beards, moustaches and sideburns change rapidly, although some cultures, such as Sikhs and Orthodox Jews, have very strict rules as to how facial hair should be worn.

Here are some examples of the many different types that have been worn in the past and some that are still worn today.

Modern beards   Medium full beard   Balbo beard

Goatee beard

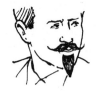
Handlebar and chin puff

Spade or Shenandoah beard

Old Dutch beard

Traditional beards

Hulihee beard

Franz Josef beard

Chin curtain beard

Modern moustaches

The military

Walrus moustache

Pencil line moustache

Handlebar moustache

Howie moustache

Square button, Hitler or Charlie Chaplin moustache

Walrus or Old Bill moustache

Adolph Menjou moustache

The major

Traditional moustaches

The general

Shermanic moustache

Painter's brush moustache

Head and face shapes

- The **oval** face shape is ideal and suits any style.
- For **round** and **square** face shapes beards need to be styled to **reduce the width** and to be cut flatter at the sides
- The **long** face shape needs to be made to appear shorter and wider. A **moustache** will help this.
- A **beard** will help to cover and minimise a small or **receding chin**.

Natural growth patterns

Facial hair grows in certain directions in the same way that scalp hair does. It mostly grows downwards and outwards, and occasionally grows in circular shapes under the chin.

Gents' traditional technique

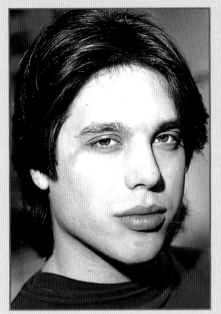

Step 1
Before: the style has completely grown out. The hair has medium texture, heavy density and very little movement.

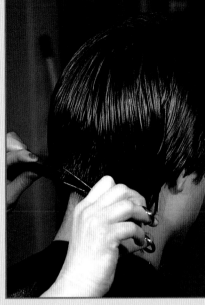

Step 2
Start to remove the bulk with scissors over comb, using large jumbo comb. Work weight up to occipital bone.

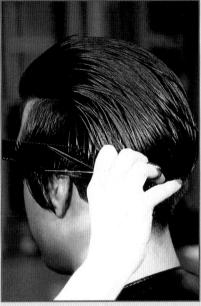

Step 3
Remove bulk from side area using large jumbo comb. Both back and sides have been cut using scissors over comb, first with jumbo comb, then cutting comb, and finally barbering combs 1 and 2.

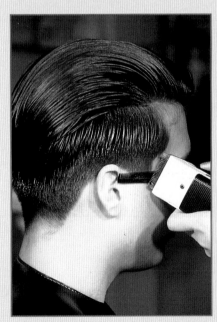

Step 4
After completing scissors over comb, for more definition and sharpness of finish use clipper over comb on both back and sides.

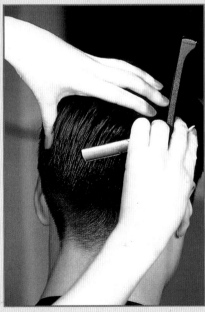

Step 5
For blending and finishing a razor may be used.

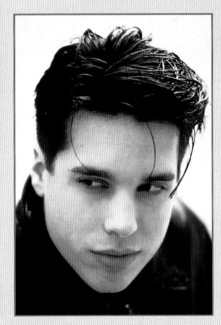

Step 6
The finished look.

Alternative finished looks for men

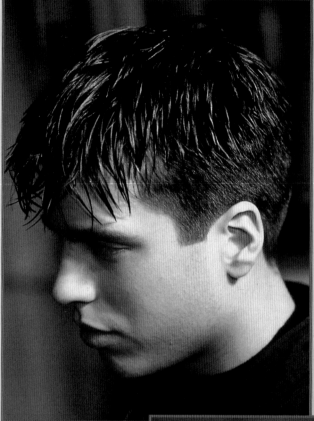

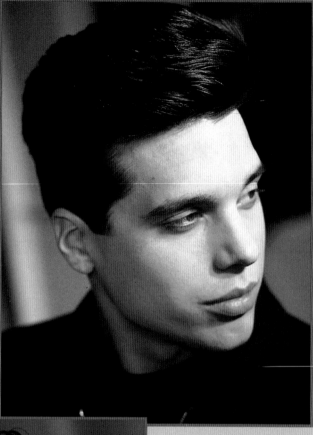

A longer version of a crew cut, using wax for a textured look.

A conventional finish, using blow-dry lotion during styling.

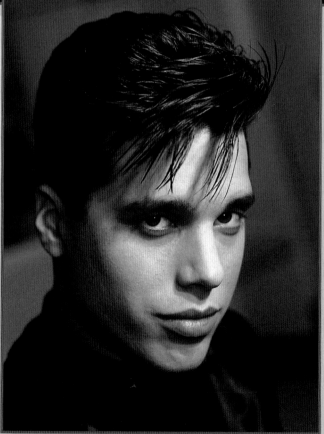

Using light men's cream for a soft finish.

Hair structures

Facial or beard hair is generally wavy or curly and much **stronger and coarser** than scalp hair.

Preparation

Gowning up

The client's clothes must be protected as normal, and both of his eyes need to be covered with a feathered-out strip of neck wool.

Positioning your client

You will need to work with your client in a **reclined** position by adjusting the barber's chair and head rest (If you don't have a barber's chair recline the client at the back wash-basin and place a towel under his neck for comfort.)

Remember
When you are cutting beard or **facial hair** the **clippings** are **very sharp and dangerous to skin and eyes**. Always protect your client as much as possible – and ask him to keep his eyes closed during cutting.

To do
■ Practise adjusting the barber's chair in all its different heights and positions – before you take your first client.

Disentangling

Disentangle the beard by combing it downwards with a wide-toothed comb.

Cutting methods

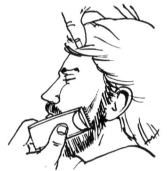

Outlining the upper part of the beard

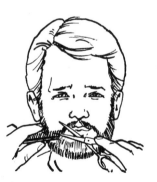

Trimming moustache and beard

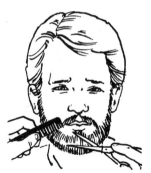

Retouch work

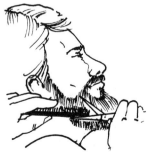

Trimming excess hair

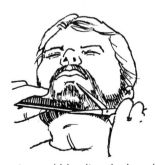

Tapering and blending the beard

Cutting a beard with scissors

Scissor over comb

Using small sections, start in the centre of the chin and work out towards the right side and then the left side. Always keep the comb and scissors **moving**. The **closer** your comb is held to the face the **shorter** the cut will be.

Clipper over comb

Cordless or rechargeable clippers are much easier to use for facial hair, because you are continually twisting and turning the clippers during cutting. **Clipper guards** are useful for **short beards** but may become entangled in longer ones. The final shape may be outlined with clippers.

Freehand cutting

The outlines of beards or moustaches are usually done freehand, without the hair being held in place with a comb or your fingers. Always **support your scissors with your first finger** when cutting a moustache to **protect the clients' lips**.

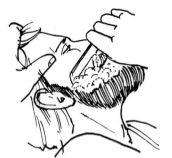

Shaving unwanted part of beard

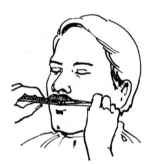

Moustache trimming

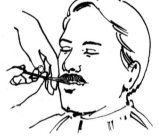

Thinning the moustache   Trimming the moustache

Razoring

A disposable open razor can be used in the same way as lining out (see p190) to remove any unwanted hair outside the desired shape.

(see p190)

Remember

Accidents can happen – re-read Chapter 10 regarding cutting yourself or the client in the salon. You are more likely to cut the client during barbering than when you are working on a female client. Use **alum powder on a small piece of damp cotton wool to stop any bleeding**, and ask the client to hold it on to the cut.

To do

■ Re-read the health and safety regulations (Chapter 10) on the safety aspects of using razors and clippers.

Finishing off

Remove all the beard clippings from your client with your neck brush then **ask the client if he is satisfied** with the result as you show him in the mirror.

Test your knowledge

1 Using drawings, photographs or illustrations, describe both traditional and current shapes of beards, moustaches and sideburns.
2 Describe the health and safety requirements regarding the use of cutting equipment.
3 What should you do if you accidentally cut your own skin?
4 What should you do if you accidentally cut your client's skin?
5 How should you dispose of used razor blades?

13 Shaving and face massage

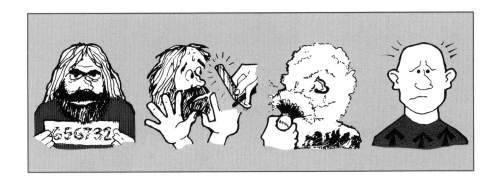

Shaving

Men's shaving and face massage is becoming more popular as today's clients need to look clean and well groomed. The art of shaving requires a steady hand, a great deal of skill and constant practice.

Safety
Using sharp razors in the salon is a risky process, so **always follow Health and Safety legislation** and local bylaw procedures.

Sharp razors must be kept **closed** and in a **safe place** (away from clients and children).

- Disposable razor blades must be **safely** disposed of (often by placing in a secure container, such as a wide-mouthed screw-topped bottle or a commercial 'sharps' container, before placing in the bin).
- Razors must be kept **sterile** (see Chapter 10) to prevent cross-infection if the client is accidentally cut (a small piece of **cotton wool dipped in alum powder is needed to stop any bleeding**). See Chapter 4 for what you should do if you accidentally cut yourself or your client.

Good communication is a vital part of shaving, you need to find out what your client requires. Does he want

- a **full face shave**?
- a **partial face shave** (does he want to keep his moustache or small beard)?

- an **outline face shave** (does he want the areas around his nape and sideburns shaved clean)?

Always consider:

- any unusual **hair growth patterns**, i.e. hair growing in lots of different directions
- any **unusual facial features** such as moles or birthmarks
- any **adverse skin conditions** such as an infection (e.g. folliculitis or impetigo), which would be spread and made worse by shaving
- hot towels (a part of shaving) should not be used on a client with **sensitive chapped or blistered skin** from heat or cold.

Tools and equipment

Barber's chair

These are hydraulically controlled, and need to be locked at the correct height and position for you to work on the client comfortably. The chair is then reclined with the head rest inserted and locked in position so that the client is comfortably laid back in the chair ready for shaving.

Steamers

Hot towels are needed to **soften and raise the facial hair** and **relax facial muscles** before shaving. Steamers are used to hold hot towels ready for shaving, and are filled with water, which heats up to provide **hot steamed towels**. If your salon does not have a steamer then the hot or cool towel can be prepared by following the diagrams below.

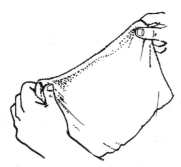

Folding a clean towel in half

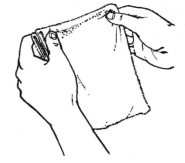

Folding towel in half again

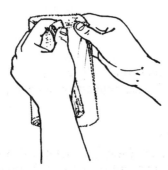

Getting ready to place towel under hot water

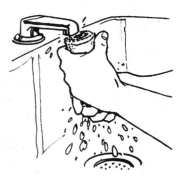

Saturating towel thoroughly with hot water

Shaving mugs and brushes

Lathering the face helps to **soften the beard** and **hold the hair** in an **upright** position. It also helps to provide a smooth, flat surface so that the razor can glide over the skin painlessly. The lather is produced from soap (which can be foam, powder, cream or liquid) and water.

A shaving mug or bowl is filled with hot water. A clean, sterile shaving brush is then immersed, removed, and a small amount of soap is placed on the bristles. The brush is then rotated vigorously (like whisking an egg), either in the bowl of the shaving mug or in a second bowl, until lather is produced.

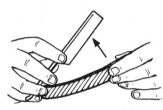

Remember

Do not use tablet soap as it would be unhygienic to use the same soap on a large number of clients.

Gowns and towels

Men's gowns are usually fastened at the back for shaving. Shaving towels are often white, and smaller than normal hairdressing towels so that they fit comfortably around the face. Paper towels, tissue or shaving squares are also used for absorbing excess lather.

Razors

Safety razors
These are used without the guard for shaving and have **disposable** blades so that each client can have their own new sterile blade for each shave.

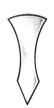

Opening razor safely

Open razors
These have **fixed blades** and there are two types.

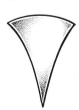

Closing razor safely

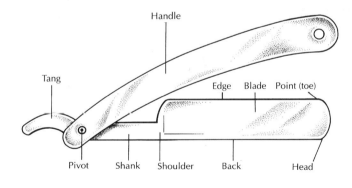

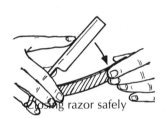

English/German hollow ground razor

English/German hollow ground
These are light, durable and pliable, but are too hard to use on sensitive skins.

French solid razor

French solid
These are made of a softer metal and are more suitable for sensitive skins (and haircutting) but have to be sharpened more often.

Honing (or setting) fixed-blade razors

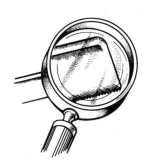

Magnified razor edge

If you magnify the edge of a razor blade you can see very fine teeth at the edge (like a tiny saw).

When razors become blunt they have to be specially sharpened with a **hone** to create a new row of teeth and be able to cut hair again.

As razors lose their sharpness quite quickly, barbers have to hone (or sharpen) their razors themselves.

A hone is a rectangular block of quarried stone. The one most frequently used is a Belgian natural hone.

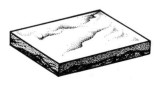

Belgian hone

To hone a hollow-ground razor

- Wipe the surface of the hone to **clean** and **free it from hair**. Place it on a tissue.
- **Lubricate** the hone with **fine oil**.
- Stroke the razor blade diagonally across the hone, leading with the sharp cutting edge. Start with the heel and finish with the toe (point). Keep equal pressure on the blade, holding it flat as you complete the movement.

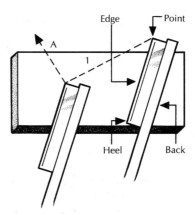

First position and stroke in honing

- Turn the razor on its back to commence the second stroke. Use your finger to turn the razor over (like rolling a pencil), **not** your wrist. As the razor is rolled over on its back, slide it upward towards the top corner of the same side. Now repeat the same diagonal movement.

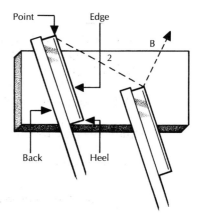

Second position and stroke in honing

- Repeat this figure-of-eight movement until the cutting edge has been restored. The oil lubricant will darken during this process as steel is removed from the blade.
- On completion, **wipe the blade along the back** with a tissue to clean it, close the blade, clean the hone and store both away safely.

To hone a French solid razor

- Clean and prepare the hone as before.
- Use a Belgian natural hone lubricated with a **fine oil**.
- The strokes should be shorter than those used for the hollow-ground razor, with only the razor edge resting, almost flat, on the hone. The stroke is more like a V shape with the razor turned on its back at the end of each stroke.

Honing a French solid razor

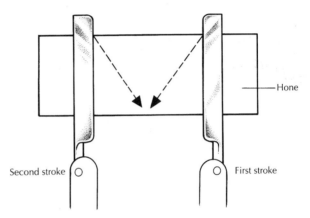

Hone

Second stroke

First stroke

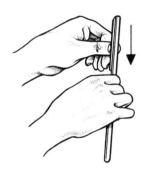

Testing razor on moistened thumbnail

Testing the razor's edge

This is done by pulling the razor across a moistened thumbnail.

- A **perfectly sharp** or keen edge will dig into the nail with a **smooth, steady grip**.
- A **blunt edge** will **pull smoothly across the nail without any dragging or cutting**.
- A **nick in the razor** will **feel uneven** when drawn across the nail.

Stropping

A razor is stropped to preserve its cutting edge between honing and setting. Stropping cleans the razor's edge and realigns the teeth, creating a **whetted edge.**

Hanging strops are used for hollow-ground razors.

Solid strops are used for French solid razors.

French or German strop

New leather strops must be smeared with oil and left to soak overnight. The canvas side of the strop should be rubbed with soap. The following day both surfaces should be rubbed with a round glass bottle until a glazed surface appears.

Stropping a hollow-ground razor

- Hang the strop on the hook then hold the free end with one hand and pull it **horizontally** out from the wall.
- Hold the razor in its straightened position with your other hand, keeping the razor shank between the first finger and thumb.
- Lie the razor flat and **stroke it** with the **back first** down the strop. When it has travelled two-thirds of the way down the strop, **turn** the razor **on its back** and repeat the stroke in the opposite direction.
- Although you will be slow to start with, your speed will increase with practice. Twelve strokes is usually sufficient to strop the razor.

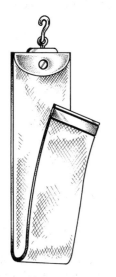

Leather and canvas strop

Remember

Never turn the razor on its edge – you could cut and split the strop and damage the razor.

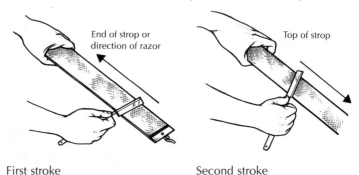

End of strop or direction of razor

Top of strop

First stroke

Second stroke

Stropping a French solid razor

The movements are the same as before but the French strop is placed in a horizontal position on a work surface. The back of the razor is lifted slightly off the strop with edge of the blade resting flat and even on the strop. The same twelve strokes are needed.

Preparing the client

- Wash your hands and nails before starting.
- Ensure that your client's beard is clean and free from grease.
- **Discuss with the client his requirements**.
- Seat the gowned client in a reclined position with a clean paper towel placed over the head rest. Make sure the client is comfortable by adjusting either the chair or gowns.

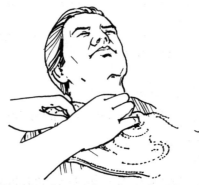

Securing the towel on the right side of the client

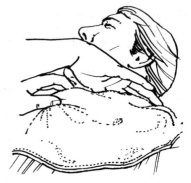

Securing the towel on the left side of the client

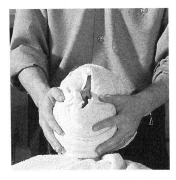

- Protect the client with a towel placed across his chest and tucked firmly into his neck.
- Check the face for any abnormalities, unusual beard growth patterns or adverse skin conditions.

Lathering

- Prepare the sterile steamed hot towel.
- Place the towel over the beard area, wrapping it over the face without covering the nose area so that the client can breathe easily.
- Strop the razor.
- Replace the cooled towel with a second hot towel.
- Prepare the brush and hot lather as previously described. Remove the second towel.
- Begin lathering the face by placing the brush on the tip of the chin and rotating it over the chin, cheeks and neck until all the beard is covered with lather. To lather the upper lip the brush is spread by placing one finger in the centre of the bristles, preventing the lather from going up the client's nose or onto his lips.
- Keep the brush hot by dipping it into the hot water. The better the lather the easier the shave.

Remember

You may cause skin irritation if the towel is too hot. Remove it and use a cooler one if it is uncomfortable for the client.

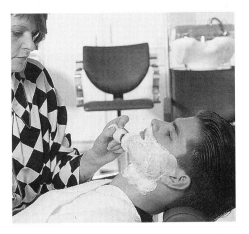

Shaving

Remember

Always stretch the skin taut during shaving.
- This holds the hair up to the razor, allowing a closer cut.
- It also helps to prevent cuts to the skin.

- It is essential that the **angle of the razor** and the **direction of the razor hold** are correct.
- The **blade** must be **wiped clean** to remove hair and lather between each razor stroke. **Always wipe the razor on its back** to prevent cutting your fingers.
- Use hot water for shaving – cold water will cause the razor to drag and be uncomfortable.

Holding the razor

There are two methods of holding the razor for shaving:

- forehand
- backhand.

You will need to practise both so that you can work at every angle of the face and neck.

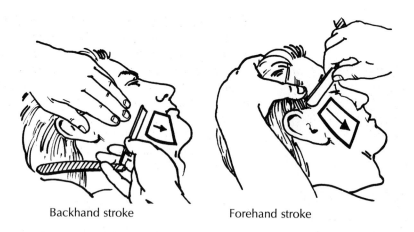

Backhand stroke   Forehand stroke

First time over shave

The first time over shave is always done in the same direction as the hair growth – with the grain of the hair.

When you are stretching the skin for this shave, place your finger **behind** the razor instead of in front of it, as it is very difficult to get a firm grip on the skin when the face is slippery with lather.

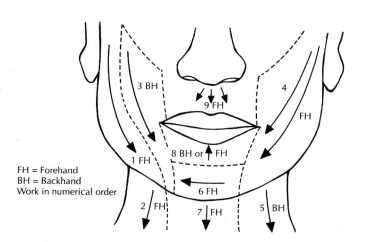

FH = Forehand
BH = Backhand
Work in numerical order

Shaving procedure: first time over

To do

■ Practise drawing the shaving movements on paper before working on a client.

Method
● Hold the razor loosely with your thumb on the blade – the actual position will vary with the different strokes. Remember to dip the razor into the warm water.
● Begin the shave on the side nearest to you. Always start by holding the dry unlathered skin at the sideburn area to prevent your fingers slipping, **pulling it taut** when you start to shave.
● Move the razor in a slicing, **scythe-like motion**, following the movements shown in the diagram.

- Each side of the face should be completely shaved before starting the other, with the centre chin section left until last.
- Incorporate each side of the upper lip area when shaving that side of the face, leaving just the centre section which is then shaved upwards while gently pressing the tip of the nose upwards to tighten the skin.
- When one side of the face has been completed, turn the client's head towards you to make it easier to shave the other side.
- To shave the point of the chin, pull the skin tight between the finger and thumb, then use the middle of the razor blade to shave across the chin.
- Finish by shaving the neck downwards.

Second time over shave

This shave is important because it ensures that the hair is cut as closely as possible giving a clean finished result. The hair is cut in an upward movement **against the growth**.

Unless the client is very dark haired with a strong beard growth, this is usually the final shave. When this is the case, it is followed by a sponge shave, which entails soaking a small sponge in hot water then dragging it across the face, closely followed by the razor.

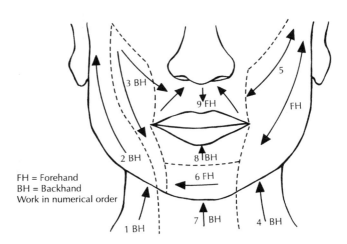

FH = Forehand
BH = Backhand
Work in numerical order

Shaving procedure: second time over

> **Remember**
>
> A right-handed barber should stand and start on the right-hand side; a left-handed one should stand and start on the left.

> **Remember**
>
> **Never shave tight curly hair too close** by shaving against the growth or grain – it is likely to cause ingrown hairs, creating swelling, infection, and possibly scarring.

> **Remember**
>
> A small piece of **damp cotton wool dipped in alum powder** should be applied to any cuts to the skin **to stop the flow** of blood. They are preferably applied by the client.

Method
- Re-lather the face.
- Start the shave at the collar area, using your fingers to hold the dry, unlathered skin.
- Move upwards in backhand strokes, completing one side of the face before starting the other (as in the diagram).
- Clean the face with a damp, warm towel or sponge, then pat dry gently with another clean towel.
- Apply a small amount of **talcum powder** to make sure that the skin is thoroughly dry.
- Finish with an **after-shave lotion**, which is an astringent and will close the pores, leaving the skin feeling fresh and clean.
- Sit the client in an upright position and check that he is satisfied with the result.

Face massage

Massage is usually carried out after shaving to aid skin elasticity, tone the facial muscles and encourage the removal of toxins. The main benefit of a face massage is to relax the client.

Before starting the massage, make sure that the client's hair and clothing are well protected from the massage cream. Prepare the equipment and make sure that your hands and nails are clean.

Method

- Steam the face with two hot towels.
- Apply the massage cream lightly over the face with stroking, spreading **effleurage** movements.
- Stroke fingers across the forehead with up and down movements.
- Manipulate your fingers across the forehead with a circular **petrissage** movement.

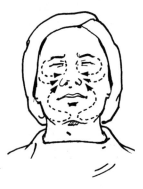

Apply cleansing cream lightly over the face with effleurage stroking, spreading and circular movements

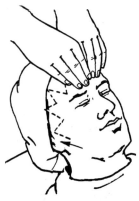

Stroke fingers across forehead with up and down movements

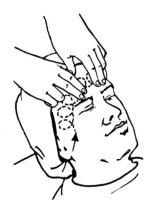

Use petrissage across forehead with a circular movement

- Stroke your fingers upwards along the side of the nose.
- Apply a circular movement over the side of the nose and use a light, stroking movement around the eyes.
- Manipulate the temples with a wide circular movement. Also manipulate the front and back of the ears with a circular **petrissage** movement.

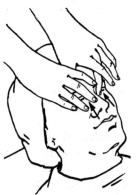

Stroke fingers upwards along the side of the nose

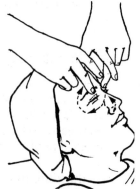

Apply a circular movement over side of nose and use a light, stroking movement around the eyes

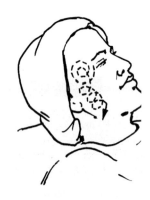

Manipulate the temples with a petrissage circular movement. Also manipulate the front and back of the ears with a circular movement

- Gently stroke both of your thumbs across the upper lip.
- Use a circular movement from the corners of the mouth, working up to the cheeks and temples, and again working along the lower jawbone from the tip of the chin to the ear.
- Stroke your fingers with an **effleurage** movement from under the chin and neck to the back of the ears and up towards the temples.

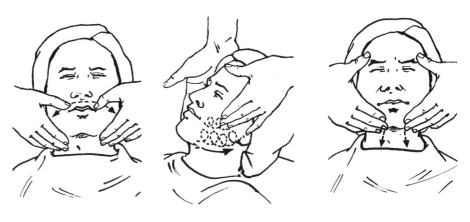

Gently stroke both thumbs across upper lip

Use a circular movement to manipulate around the jaw

Manipulate fingers from under chin and neck to back of ears and up to temples

- Complete the treatment with another hot towel followed by a cool towel. An astringent may be used to close the pores and tighten up the skin.

Finishing products

- Talcum powder may be used to soothe and dry the skin helping to reduce the effect of oily, shiny skin.
- Face creams will soothe and moisturise and help to correct dry skin conditions.
- After-shave lotions will close the skin's pores and reduce both skin irritation and the risk of infection. They act both as an astringent and a mild antiseptic, leaving a pleasant smell.
- After-shave balms will soothe the skin as they contain conditioners and leave a pleasant smell. They do not sting, unlike after-shave lotions.

Vibro massage

Remember
Use the vibro gently and carefully. If it feels too strong for the client then use the attachments over your hand.

This is a mechanical massage that can be used instead of a hand massage. It produces very strong **tapotement** (tapping) movements, which are only suitable for fleshy areas of skin. It can be very uncomfortable for the client when used on bony areas such as the forehead and jawline, and it must **never** be used around the eyes or on the nose.

Use the vibro in the same order and in the same direction as in the diagrams for the hand massage.

Sit the client upright and check that he is satisfied with the result.

Massage – movement	Effect
Effleurage – stroking	soothing and relaxing
Petrissage – deep kneading	stimulates muscles and nerves improving the circulation
Tapotement – tapping	tones the muscles, breaks down fatty deposits and increases the blood flow to the skin
Vibro massage – mechanical tapping	tones the muscles, breaks down fatty deposits and increases the blood flow to the skin

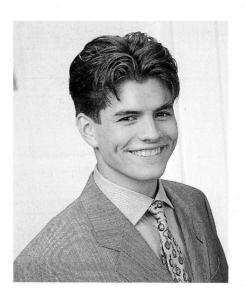

Test your knowledge

1 Describe the health and safety requirements regarding the use of razors.
2 How should you dispose of used razor blades?
3 What should you do if you accidentally cut your own skin?
4 What should you do if you accidentally cut your client's skin?
5 Why should the skin be stretched taut during shaving?
6 Name two finishing products that may be used after shaving and describe their uses.
7 Why is it important to consult with the client throughout the shaving process?
8 Describe how hot and cool towels are used and the effects they have on the skin.
9 Name and describe each type of face massage technique.

Index